HEALING
THE
HEALER

What Fifty Years as a Physician/Psychiatrist While

Having Multiple Sclerosis Taught Me About Healing

HEALER
THE
HEALER

What Fifty Years as a Physician/Psychiatrist While

Having Multiple Sclerosis Taught Me About Healing

SUMTER CARMICHAEL M.D.

(Belle Sumter Miller Carmichael Coleman)

Birmingham, Alabama

For information about this title or to order other books
and/or electronic media, contact the publisher:
bellesumter@bellsouth.net

Cover and interior design by The Book Cover Whisperer:
OpenBookDesign.biz

979-8-9869814-7-5 Paperback
979-8-9869814-6-8 Hardcover
979-8-9869814-8-2 eBook

Printed in the United States of America

FIRST EDITION

CONTENTS

Introduction i

PART ONE 1

Chapter One: The Destructive Nature of Diagnosis 3

Chapter Two: My Introduction to Medicine 13

Chapter Three: Lessons From the South 29

Chapter Four: A Dark Period: Multiple Sclerosis, Divorce,
and Male Bullying. 40

Chapter Five: Who Are the Charlatans? And What I Learned
From Orthomolecular Psychiatry 53

Chapter Six: What Drugs and Addiction Taught Me 62

Chapter Seven: What MS Taught Me About Chronic Illness 71

Chapter Eight: What Injury Taught Me About Recovery
from Pain 79

Chapter Nine: What Overdoing It Taught Me About
Managing Limitations 88

Chapter Ten: Giving Back—Learning How Helping Others
is a Constructive Way to Help Yourself. 96

Chapter Eleven: Revisiting My Diagnosis and the Role of
the Doctor 109

PART TWO 121

Chapter Twelve: Chronic Pain Became the Vehicle for
Understanding the Importance of Alternative or
Natural Therapies: The Role of Depression and
Other Emotions in a Medical Setting 123

Chapter Thirteen: So, What About Food?. 138

Chapter Fourteen: Understanding How Homeopathy and
Other Natural or Alternative Medical Therapies
Became Discredited 149

Chapter Fifteen: History Of Medicine's War on Natural
Therapies. 156

Chapter Sixteen: American Medical Association Enters the
Medical Drama 163

Chapter Seventeen: Rockefeller Medicine: How the Actions of One Man Changed the Direction of Medicine in America 167

Chapter Eighteen: How Money Dominates AMA Resistance to Natural Therapies 172

Chapter Nineteen: The Power of the Mind to Influence the Body: Emotions and Healing; Enter the Placebo Effect 182

Chapter Twenty: The Truth About Healing and Spirituality. 198

Chapter Twenty-One: Embracing Alternative Therapies: Where We Are Today In the War to Discredit Natural Therapy 207

PART THREE 215

Chapter Twenty-Two: How Using Science as the Only Standard to Understand the Patient is Limiting What Doctors Have to Offer 217

Chapter Twenty-Three: The Opiate Epidemic: Are Doctors Making Us Worse? This is What You Need to Know to Assess and Safely Treat Chronic Pain 229

Chapter Twenty-Four: The Future of Medicine: Genuine Healthcare for America: How Racism Has Limited Healthcare and Education for Everyone 244

Author's Comments and Acknowledgements. 259

Author's Biography 261

The practice of medicine is an art, not a trade; a calling,
not a business; a calling in which your heart will be
exercised equally with your head."
— WILLIAM OSLER

"It is reasonable to expect the doctor to recognize that
science may not have all the answers to problems
of health and healing."
— NORMAN COUSINS

Introduction

Death and disability are parts of life. But we don't have to embrace disaster. Our body is wired to survive, to heal. From the trauma of the birth canal to your last breath, your unconscious is working to keep you safe, mend your injuries, and lead you to healthful living and recovery.

This book is the narrative of what I discovered about healing in the course of being a doctor/psychiatrist for over fifty years, teaching medical students and young doctors for over thirty years, all the while having multiple sclerosis since age 30. I want each reader to understand the events that have influenced my thinking and helped me persevere. To recover from injury, I learned what works best for those faced with chronic pain and depression.

In the pain clinic I established for the poor in 2003, I found that neither the physicians nor their patients knew what to do for chronic pain, and how depression played its part. That prompted me to write my first two books, published in 2012. *HEAL: A Psychiatrist's Inspiring Story of What It Takes to Recover from Chronic Pain, Depression and Addiction . . . And What Stands in the Way,* and *HEAL THYSELF: What You Can Do to Recover from Chronic Pain, Depression and Addiction.*

In those books, I talked only peripherally about having MS, and I still had many unanswered questions about healing that I have resolved in the ensuing years. In this book, I plan to talk about how I survived MS, delve into the blind spots in my profession, and unravel questions about healing.

I also want to consider what it means to be a doctor, how I discovered the truth about healing, and why, at times, modern medicine fails us all.

I include my tale of how I learned about addiction and the use of opiates, the importance of the doctor-patient relationship, and what is needed to recover from chronic pain. I had to find these elements for myself as I had never been taught these things as part of my training.

In the course of learning about chronic pain, I discovered many alternative therapies and where the blind spots about these therapies in my profession originated. I even discovered why assessing pain as the fifth vital sign is encouraging addiction and training patients to take pills for their pain instead of looking for other ways to manage their discomfort, some known for centuries.

Over the years, I learned about the importance of food and nutrition and why nutrition is not routinely taught to doctors as part of their training. Finally, science has teased out the source of some of our most pressing mysteries, like why exercise is such a powerful tool, how the placebo effect works, and the cause of hysteria, all of which I will discuss in detail.

In my first year of psychiatric training, when relatively few women were in practice, I was bullied by a group of male doctors. In this book, I am able to tell that story and how it fits in with the dominant medical profession's attacks on natural therapies, a battle that goes back centuries.

Finally, I discovered more recently how medicine had become the lackey of the pharmaceutical industry, how medicine became a fee-for-service system that makes money for medical practitioners, insurance companies, and the pharmaceutical industry, but does not address the health needs of American citizens, even the very rich.

In the last chapter, I described the weaknesses in the healthcare system exposed by the COVID-19 virus, including systemic racism. Throughout the book, I discover the power of the unconscious to drive events for good and for ill.

Part One is my personal story of discovery about how I survived MS and what adversity taught me. Part Two will demonstrate how I discovered what facilitates healing and where American medicine went off track. Part Three describes some current ills and looks at future of the profession.

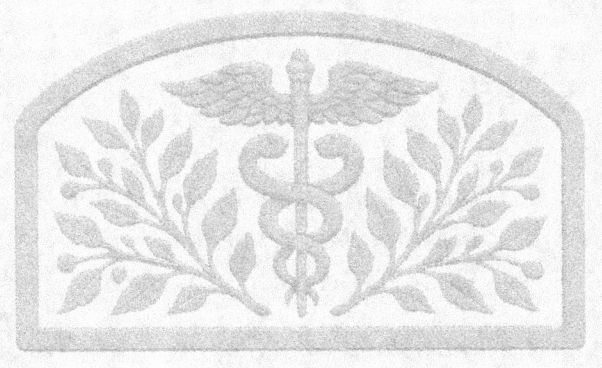

PART ONE

*"He is the best physician who is the most
ingenious inspirer of hope."*
— SAMUEL TAYLOR COLERIDGE

*"You have to understand what they are worried about,
what their fears are, what they are trying to do? If we
don't engage with them that way, it doesn't
matter what technology we use."*
— ROY ROSIN, CHIEF INNOVATION OFFICER,
PENN MEDICINE

*"There is only one cardinal rule: One must
always listen to the patient."*
— OLIVER SACKS

CHAPTER ONE

The Destructive Nature of Diagnosis

In 1968, I had my first symptom of multiple sclerosis, one of the dread diseases of young adulthood. MS is a devastating illness that has the potential to cause the loss of all functions as a person: movement, sensation, and even the ability to think or feel joy. By 1988, I was asked to join the Medical Advisory Board of the MS Society. There, I met Dr. Eric Martin, the new chairman of Neurology and a specialist in MS. Dr. Martin was starting a clinic to evaluate potential MS patients. With few definitive tests to identify the disease, the clinic was set up to evaluate difficult-to-diagnose patients and help those with severe diseases that were difficult to manage. Dr. Martin was eager for me to help him and the other neurologists in his Clinic. I agreed to leave my psychiatric practice one morning a week to volunteer at the Clinic.

Working with patients in this clinic, I thought I was one of the lucky ones—I thought I had already survived MS. While my symptoms might fluctuate, I thought MS was no longer a threat to my survival or my ability to function fully as a person.

Still, when Interferon first appeared in 1994, I thought I should see if it would benefit me. Looking back, I can see how denial had helped me live with this dangerous illness and how blessed I had been to be doing as well as I was.

When Interferon appeared, I asked Dr. Martin if he would see me as a patient to determine if I would benefit from taking the new medicine. That is how I happened to be sitting in his waiting room on a brisk fall afternoon, waiting for his answer.

Dr. Eric Martin was the University's leading MS specialist, and I knew he had great respect for me as a psychiatrist. When the University had asked him to head the department of Psychiatry as well as Neurology, he told me he would only do it if I ran the Psych department for him! But as I waited to hear what he was going to say about putting me on medication for life, I could not help feeling a sense of dread mixed with terror.

The nurse called me into his office. As he was every Tuesday in the MS Clinic, Dr. Martin was dressed in a long white coat with his bag of neurology tools in his pocket. He pointed to a seat. His face was impassive as he pulled out my chart to look at my test results.

"Your tests show you have chronic-progressive multiple sclerosis," he said. "You have had optic neuritis in both eyes, in addition to problems with your gait. Your hearing has been affected by the disease as well."

His words could not have hit me harder if I were learning I had MS for the first time. Of course, I already knew I had multiple sclerosis. At some level, I'd known from my very first twinge that it was probably multiple sclerosis, but since working in the MS clinic, I thought that I was doing really well.

I had already given Dr. Martin my history at our first appointment ten days earlier. At that first interview, he never asked me how

I could be doing so well after twenty-five years, how long it had been since my last MS episode, what I was doing with my life, or how much I was exercising.

All he did was ask questions from what sounded like a disability scale, and by that measurement, other than using a cane sometimes, I was perfectly functional—100% functional! I had a limp and some sensory symptoms, but that was all. And in spite of how I was doing, he was telling me I had the worst kind of multiple sclerosis? Chronic Progressive MS?

As Dr. Martin started to speak again, I forced myself to listen. "Unfortunately, at this time, we're only studying the effects of Interferon on patients with relapsing-remitting multiple sclerosis (the best kind of MS, if you have to have it)." He took a breath. "If anything else comes along, I will let you know."

I was stunned. Why is he telling me I have the worst kind of multiple sclerosis if he has nothing to offer me? How is this supposed to help me? Why is he telling me this at all? All I came for was to find out if this new medicine to treat MS would be helpful to me. He did not need to tell me more than that.

"So, you won't be giving Interferon to me?" I asked, taken aback.

"Not at this time," he said before he trailed off into a discussion of other drugs coming down the pipeline. "I can give you a call if something becomes available."

Suddenly, I could not hear him anymore because I was suffused with anger. Why give me the worst diagnosis possible if you have nothing to offer me?

I thought to myself, "Diagnoses are for doctors to develop treatment plans, insurance companies to pay, and disability determinations, not for making patients feel worse. After all, the first axiom in medicine is, "Do no harm!" Diagnoses should be given to patients only if they accomplish something positive for the patient or point the way to future action.

The Healing Power of Belief

DOCTORS MUST UNDERSTAND THAT what people believe about themselves determines how well they do. In a 2019 scientific study, patients were told the opposite of their test results to see if how well they did was reflected in their actual numbers or if what they believed determined how well they did. As it turned out, the numbers had little to do with how patients fared. The biggest factor in how patients did was in what they believed about themselves.

Psychologist Alia Crum at Stanford studied the effect of telling house cleaners who did not exercise that their work gave them all the necessary exercise to keep them in peak health. He found that knowledge alone made them healthier.

It made me think of two patients I had seen as a resident physician in the 1970s. Both patients had a deadly leukemia that would lead to their deaths in the near future. Their lab values were identical.

One patient believed God had a hand in his disease and had given him this trial so he could be useful to others. His family and members of his church surrounded him, and despite the terrible diagnosis, he remained positive about his outcome. The other man, however, felt hopeless and died alone the very next day.

As a psychiatrist, I felt that Dr. Martin failed to have any empathy for my situation. Despite my working relationship with him and the respect I knew he had for me as a medical colleague, Dr. Martin was acting as if he did not understand how he could help me.

He could not get past his standard approach with patients—that is, to test, diagnose, and treat—in order to fulfill the needs of his study. He did not give me anything that would benefit me. It never occurred to him that running tests and making diagnoses did not make sense if they wouldn't help me.

Yes, I already knew I had multiple sclerosis. If Dr. Martin couldn't make my life better, his obligation was to be as positive and encouraging as possible. Had he listened to my history, he would have already known I was not right for his study. I had not had a new MS episode in so long that he would have had no way of knowing whether the medicine was doing anything positive.

Beyond that, he could have told me that I was doing too well to take Interferon, which was true for people early in their illness who were having lots of episodes. He could have told me he did not even know if Interferon would benefit someone like me. He could have made me feel positive about not being part of his study, which would have made me sick for days every week. He could have told me to keep doing whatever I was doing because it seemed to be helping me. He never even showed any interest at all in what I might be doing myself, which was slowing the progression of my disease.

I already knew, from seeing MS patients for depression in my office, that taking Interferon was a great boon to those who were newly diagnosed with multiple sclerosis. Knowing that the MS was being treated, each of my patients felt a great weight lifted. My patients with MS were less depressed and more optimistic, even though they were sick for several days every week from taking the Interferon. They did not seem to mind being sick often since it meant to them that their multiple sclerosis would not get any worse.

Before Dr. Martin told me that I had the worst kind of MS: (chronic-progressive multiple sclerosis)[1] And had shaken my con-

1   Mult ple sclerosis is generally divided into two common types: relapsing-remitting (RRMS), which comes and goes in a matter of weeks or months, and chronic-

fidence, I really believed the MS was under control. After all, I had not had a new symptom in several years.

In fact, looking at the patients I was seeing in the MS clinic at that time, I believed I had already survived MS. I knew I would always have the old damage that would affect my gait and other parts of my body, but I felt safe that it would not get too much worse.

At least I won't get sick from treatment several days a week, I thought. Suddenly, I was relieved he had not wanted me to take Interferon. Who wants to be dragged into the medical circus anyway? Still, I thought, "How could he leave me hanging like that?" I continued to fume to myself for some time.

That experience with Dr. Martin confirmed my decision to stay away from neurologists who apparently had nothing helpful to offer me and just made me feel bad. I did go see a neurologist or my internist whenever I had a new symptom that I did not understand. I wanted to be sure I did not have something else that required treatment.

But I turned down most MRIs since I already knew I had multiple sclerosis. In fact, over the years, I turned down a lot of tests and medicines ordered by other doctors that I did not think would help me and might make me worse. My experience with doctors had taught me that their vision tended to be limited to their narrow way of looking at illness and treatment, the so-called bio-medical model, and all too often did not include my concerns or needs.

---

progressive (CPMS), which gets progressively worse over time. CPMS basically falls into three types. 1) Primary-progressive MS occurs in about 10% of patients with multiple sclerosis. These people get worse slowly from the beginning. 2) Progressive-relapsing MS, which rapidly gets worse from the start, and represents 5% of patients with MS. 3) The most common type is secondary-progressive MS (SPMS). SPMS occurs in 80% of those who start off with relapsing-remitting MS.

The Importance of Understanding the Patient's Experience

EVEN IN MY YOUTH, I sensed that my role as a physician was more than making a diagnosis and plugging in some medicine. By staying focused on the patient's concerns, the doctor is more apt to understand what the patient's problem actually was at that moment, so he could make the right assessment for this patient at that particular time.

At least, the doctor could keep the focus on understanding that the patient's experience was central to helping patients with their own concerns. How else can doctors bolster the patient's recovery? Otherwise, they risk getting caught up in their own drama and interests, making a diagnosis, and plugging in some drug or other concrete intervention. They often fail to see how the patient's psyche plays a major role in dealing with illness and taking steps to get better.

Also, I knew that psychiatrists generally tended to be more perceptive than other doctors. As a trainee in psychiatry, I had wondered when I would begin to have that second sight psychiatrists seemed to have. It took me until my senior year as a resident-in-training to realize psychiatrists know more than other doctors, not because they're more discerning than other doctors, but because patients tell them more.

Psychiatrists are trained to elicit information and really listen to what patients have to say. They understand that unraveling the cause of patients' emotions and behavior, and not just their physical symptoms, gives them the best chance of understanding what is needed for this patient at that moment in time, and facilitating movement.

That understanding guides the physician to make the correct interventions for each patient. In addition, psychiatrists were also trained to recognize their own biases and conflicts, so these do not interfere with understanding and giving patients what they need.

In today's bio-medical-without-psyche world, talking with patients to determine how psychosocial issues[2] affect their health is not the focus of today's medical practitioner, in part because it takes too much time, and time is money, but also because limiting one's focus to concrete issues is a major way doctors deal with their own anxiety. It's an unconscious defense against anxiety, something we'll return to later.

Advantages of Being a Woman in Medicine

THERE ARE SOME ADVANTAGES to being an outsider in medicine, as I was—both as a woman and as a patient. Being a woman may have given me more empathy with patients and more flexibility in trying to understand what was going on with them. I also felt freer to try non-traditional approaches to help my patients, like using meditation, exercise, and dietary changes to treat chronic pain, rather than looking for a pain pill or injection to fix the problem.

As an outsider, I observed the profession from a perspective that challenged what I'd been taught during my training as a doctor. It may have allowed me to see where standard medicine or standard psychiatry has strayed from the ideal path.

Medical Education is a Process of Indoctrination

Too often, I saw medical students trained to judge situations by preconceived biases. Yes, medical education is a process of indoctrination. Medical students are trained to evaluate information in a routine and systematic way. There is, of course, a benefit in having

2   Emotional, social, and spiritual issues.

a routine and even a benefit in having checklists to ensure nothing important is forgotten or left out.

But without a mechanism to shift to another paradigm to evaluate what else may be contributing to a problem or what else may help patients, physicians tend to overlook some of the most important tools available to them.

My lessons began in 1960, when I entered medical school.

"A good physician treats the disease, the great physician treats the patient who has the disease."
— UNKNOWN

"A wise man should consider that health is the greatest of human blessings, and learn how by his own thought to benefit from his illnesses."
— HIPPOCRATES

"Each patient carries his own doctor inside him."
— NORMAN COUSINS, ANATOMY OF AN ILLNESS

CHAPTER TWO

My Introduction to Medicine

Entering medical school in 1960, I believed medicine to be the most honorable of all professions, practiced by people dedicated to making a difference in their patients' lives. I saw this in the doctors who trained me and in the doctors whom I encountered along the way. I was part of a medical world dedicated to making medical treatment better.

In the 1960s, thanks to vaccines, we were heady with our advances against polio and other infectious diseases. It seemed as if we were going to eradicate all infectious diseases from the planet in my lifetime. I didn't really understand, back then, how the myths we tell ourselves about the past override everything we do.

Little did we imagine that our success with vaccines would erase our memories of plague and pestilence and of how many had lost their lives that way. We could not imagine the advent of diseases like AIDS or COVID-19, though we should have based on past experience.

Little did we understand in the 1960s how human dynamics—"politics"—could alter the future direction of medicine as they do for religion, not always for the better.

Discrimination Against Women

ENTERING MEDICINE AT A time when discrimination against women in the profession was high, I experienced prejudice in many ways, both in New York, where I went to medical school, and in Birmingham, Alabama, where I ended up training to become a psychiatrist. Today, there are so many women in medicine that one would think sexism has ended, but no. It has simply become a subterranean part of the culture.

Today, in the South, my very fine doctor-friends encourage their own daughters who are interested in medicine to become nurses, not doctors like themselves. And the Catholic priest at my grand-daughter's school teaches girls that their job is to have children, not pursue a career, not recognizing that not all women have a man to support them throughout life.

The reality in today's world, especially in the South, is that some women are trained to become wives and mothers while others are encouraged to pursue intellectual interests for themselves.

I was born to an upper-class family, impoverished by the Depression in the 1930s. On the one hand, I expected all the world's opportunities to be open to me, so I only applied to the best medical schools, but I also believed marriage was the most important decision I would make in my life.

My father urged me to have a career. His father had died when he was twenty, and he had had to give up his inheritance to support his two older unmarried sisters. He knew firsthand the importance of having girls trained to care for themselves.

From an early age, I was drawn to Jesus and the church, and I was confirmed in the Episcopal Church at age nine. I might have pursued the ministry had I not been a girl, so medicine seemed a sacred choice in its place.

My desire to help humanity as a doctor found me in high school when I imagined myself going off to deepest Africa with a dedicated man to minister to the sick and poor. Who would have thought that an interest in psychiatry and the discrimination I endured as a female in medicine would ultimately lead me to treat the poor at the local county hospital in my fifties and make me more attuned to the shortcomings in my profession?

When the day came, I applied to all the best medical schools. Stanford accepted my application, but it was a five-year program, and since I would have to pay my own way, I decided to work for a year and reapply to East Coast schools the following year.

The National Institutes of Health (NIH) was eager to hire me as a mathematician since I had just graduated from Stanford with honors in math. So, I headed to Washington, where I shared an apartment with one of my college roommates across the river from Georgetown in Virginia.

With graduation money from my grandparents, I bought a bright-red Austin Healey Sprite secondhand. Each day, I drove through Georgetown to Bethesda in Maryland, tooling along. (Periodically, I had to stop to lift the hood and screw in the wolf whistle, which would work its way out after a few uses.)

I could not believe my good fortune living in Washington, D.C., where I had spent my early years before being moved about with my father by the Navy. Once settled in, I began writing to East Coast medical schools to apply for the following year.

Within a month, I got a call from Cornell Medical College in New York City. "We just got your application for next year," the Dean said. "One of the students in the freshman class has come down with mono. If you want to come this year, there's a place for you."

I was stunned. It's true that I started at Stanford in pre-med, but I soon switched to being a music major. I switched again to math at the beginning of my junior year because it was the easiest program for me to complete in two years.

But when the "love of my life" went to medical school and married another woman, I realized that the medical profession was my true direction and turned my sights back to medicine. With classes only in elementary botany and the classification of flowering plants, plus organic chemistry, I applied to the best medical schools in the country, including Cornell.

I realized that this call from Cornell was my chance, and I jumped at it. I sold my Austin Healey and soon left for New York. I never stopped to think how I would pay my way. I would have to get a job.

This was in the 1960s, when television programming was limited, and families were able to keep their children ignorant of the world until they were old enough or mature enough to handle the realities of life. I used to say in jest that I had to go to medical school to find out about those "things" ladies were not supposed to know.

My aristocratic grandmother had been schooled in Dresden, Germany, where her wealthy parents took their children to live in 1898. She later married a naval officer and had her own adventures in Hawaii and Haiti.

After my mother's birth in 1905, she survived a year of illness caused by childbed fever, but she did not mention it in the autobiography she wrote after her hundredth birthday.

When I asked her about the omission, she said, "Ladies don't talk about such 'things.' Not in a memoir." I was torn between wanting to follow the path of the women in my family and wanting to strike out on my own adventures. And going to medical school at Cornell was my chance.

Due to my interest in the Church, I planned to pursue psychiatry, the field closest to being a minister in my mind. Thanks to my proclivity for math, I also hoped to do research. Being a whiz at math meant I had that kind of mind, didn't it?

Only later did I realize that math is an intuitive function. My strength was in intuition, not deductive reasoning. I still dreamed of following some wonderful man into darkest Africa as a medical missionary, so I had not fully escaped the message and training that my job as a woman was to please a man and follow him, not go my own way.

In the end, that meant when I decided to marry, rather than go to Mass General at Harvard for my residency in psychiatry, I stayed in Birmingham, where my husband was to train in neurology, even though there was no psychiatry.

Nevertheless, in 1964, still possessing the brashness of youth, I did not doubt that I could do anything I set my mind to. And since I had not yet found that elusive man to follow, I was free to have adventures of my own. I was bold, certainly, but also naive about the world. I had a lot to learn about people and how the world, especially the world of medicine, works. But what an adventure!

Being the daughter of a naval officer, I had traveled around the country and even lived in England and France while those countries were still recovering from World War II. I had been to both private and public schools with all kinds of people, so I felt as grounded as any young person heading off to New York to experience the rigors of medical school.

It just didn't occur to me that being a woman would be an issue.

As the elder of two girls and the daughter and granddaughter of navy wives, I never considered being female a problem.

Medical School

WHEN I ARRIVED AT Cornell, school had already been in session for a week. My parents drove me from their home in West Orange, New Jersey, to New York and the dorm on 69th Street and York Avenue across from New York Hospital. Sitting majestically on the East River, New York Hospital dominates the landscape. My room on the second floor for women looked out on the Rockefeller Institute across the way and beyond it, the 59th Street Bridge sparkling in the sunlight. Could I really be here? Could I really be in medical school?

Reporting to the dean's office, I got my schedule and a tour of the facilities. The secretary took me around New York Hospital's impressive lobby and showed me the Victorian-era lecture halls where I would have classes. I did not yet know about J.D. Rockefeller's role in building these facilities and fundamentally reshaping my profession at the dawn of the Twentieth century.

As I walked the halls, I was too caught up in the feeling of awe at following the thousands of medical students who had preceded me and the honor of being part of a sacred tradition. It seemed I had walked into another life.

Focused on my own survival, I asked about job opportunities and was given a list to choose from. The first job I found was as a night watchman at the psychiatric hospital. I would answer the phone in the lobby from six p.m. to midnight. The doors would be locked. I could study while I worked.

The second job I came across was serving as a mathematician for an epidemiologist at the Rockefeller Institute. With no such thing as a calculator or adding machine yet available to anyone, I would calculate statistics in my head. Both were perfect jobs for me.

The next day, in anatomy class, Dr. Swan, head of the department, introduced me to my classmates and encouraged them to make me feel at home. I was one of seven women in the freshman class.

This was the first time Cornell had had more than one or two women in a medical school class since the 1920s, when many women entered the profession. We eventually graduated with sixty-seven students, ten of them women. Several of the men dropped out, but three women transferred in from other places during our junior year.

Thanks to the small number of students and the classes we all took together, medical school was a little like being back in boarding school. We lived together, ate meals together, and went to the same lectures together. In such close quarters, I found young men could be as silly as a bunch of girls, gossiping and carrying on.

On my first day, one of the men charged ahead of me through the door, snarling at me that I had given up my right to be treated like a woman by going to medical school. This was my first exposure to discrimination for being a woman.

In general, as I got to know my classmates, I found them to be good comrades. They occasionally made jokes about the girls not belonging there, but I did not sense real hostility behind their comments. And in some ways, being a woman was an advantage.

After our first anatomy exam, Dr. Swan summoned me to his office. I asked around and learned that no one else had gotten such a message. As our meeting approached, I grew very nervous. Surely, I can't be the only person to fail the first exam.

Dr. Swan was very kind and solicitous. It turned out I was the only freshman working while attending school. I did not know freshmen were not supposed to work. He sent me to discuss my finances with the dean.

The dean took a look at my file and said, "You're in luck. We have lots of students who need financial help, but we have limited resources for the men. But there's a lot of money to assist women students. Just tell us what you need."

I did not quit my jobs, but the school refunded my tuition and gave me a full scholarship to cover all my expenses. I figured out a budget, asking for the bare minimum. I bought my clothes from the secondhand stores on Second Avenue and drank milk instead of Coca-Cola to make the most of my food money.

I was so proud of being frugal that I wore one blouse with a V-neck, backward and forward, under my little white coat. That way, I had a high neckline and a V-neckline with one blouse.

To supplement my diet, I made yogurt from a teaspoon of live-culture yogurt in hot tap water in my room. Looking back, I realize that may not have been very sanitary since we had no refrigeration, but my roommate and I got away with it. The only problem it caused was in the bacteriology lab. We were told to culture our mouths to see what bacteria occur naturally. All we could find in our own throats was *lactobacillus*, the organism in yogurt.

My junior year, I went back to see the dean about money. I told him I wanted to buy some clothes and go skiing over break. He looked at my budget, said I had never asked for enough money in the first place, and gave me more than I requested. Even though being a woman inspired periodic discrimination, it did have big advantages!

Bellevue Hospital

DURING MY JUNIOR YEAR, I encountered actual patients for the first time. Almost immediately, I discovered what a difference I could make in their lives, even with my level of training. I was especially thrilled to find myself assigned to Bellevue Hospital for my senior rotation in surgery.

Since I would be spending many nights on call at Bellevue, I was assigned a room there for the duration. Classes still took place at Cornell on 69th Street, so I either rode my bicycle back and forth or hitchhiked on the East River Drive. Many of my fellow classmates also hitchhiked.

Wearing our short white coats, which identified us as medical students, we would stand by the side of the road, waiting for a ride. Hitchhiking would have seemed like a dangerous occupation anywhere else, but here, protected by the cloak of youth and medical ID, I felt safe with those giving us a ride.

Once, I even got a ride in a police van. Most often, it was the poor who gave us a ride. Someone I knew got a ride from a yacht docked in the East River near Bellevue, a spot I revisited years later, sailing from Newport to Annapolis.

My introduction to Bellevue was a tour of the facility when I first arrived. At the emergency area, I was ushered into a huge, high-ceilinged room with patients seated around the edges, separated by screens. "Everyone has to come in here first and be deloused," the tour guide explained. It was a little unnerving seeing these facilities from the last century.

Rebuilt during the Victorian era, Bellevue was a world away from the gleaming halls and rooms of the majestic New York Hospital. New York Hospital was the place for the wealthy and connected, while Bellevue was for the poor and derelict, as it had been since it was first built in 1660.

We hear about the differences in healthcare today between the rich and privileged and the poor and minorities, but in the past, these distinctions were even more extreme. Wealthy hospitals like New York Hospital would not only turn away despised people like the Irish when they first came to the US, but they also turned away those with serious diseases or infections, keeping their own facilities pristine.

Even Christian hospitals distinguished between the "worthy poor" and the "undeserving poor." I had always assumed that Christian facilities would minister to the most destitute, but I soon learned this wasn't the case. These institutions catered to wealthier classes who had fallen on hard times, like widows and orphans, leaving the dregs of society either to be abandoned or to be cared for by the state—in this case, Bellevue Hospital.

The real difference between hospitals was in nursing care. Since the 17th, 18th, and even 19th centuries, medical care has involved heroic measures in all allopathic hospitals. Even when used to treat those who could pay, these 'heroic measures'[3] often hastened death.

Bellevue appears to be the first medical establishment set up in the American colonies to help the poor. The Dutch built a small infirmary on the site in 1660, but it was not until 1736 that the British built the first almshouse for the poor and insane.

Due to the influx of European refugees into New York City during the 17th and 18th centuries, New York became a hub for diseases, with measles, influenza, scarlet fever, diphtheria, and yellow fever outbreaks. In addition, scarcely a decade went by in the 1700s without an outbreak of smallpox, killing as many as five hundred people each time.

Edward Jenner's discovery of vaccination reduced the threat of smallpox by 1800, but by then, yellow fever was becoming an even

---

3   Phlebotomy, purging, medicines with lead, mercury and arsenic.

more significant threat. Brought to the Americas by slave ships from Africa, the mosquito Aedes aegypti transmitted yellow fever, and the disease killed half the people it infected.

Some of these deaths were hastened by the treatment known as phlebotomy, or bloodletting, which had been popular with allopathic doctors since ancient times. Phlebotomy is thought to have brought a death sentence to our first president, George Washington. Standard medical treatment in the West has always had the potential to worsen patients. Up through the 19th century, doctors were still bleeding their patients and using medicine that contained mercury, lead, and even arsenic.

In 1876, Joseph Lister introduced antiseptic surgery to this country at Bellevue Hospital as a way to prevent fatal infections after surgery. Many doctors were skeptical of the need for such a process at the time, even though they were losing two-thirds of all surgery patients to bacterial infections after their operations. With extreme sanitation, these deaths ceased.

By the time I arrived at Bellevue Hospital in 1964, the hospital was an anachronism, with its thirty-five-bed wards, antiquated elevators, fitful electrical system, and no air conditioning. In the summer, the windows facing the East River were opened, and surgical procedures had to be canceled if the temperature got too high. A shortage of nurses meant we might have to wait in the middle of a surgery while the next shift of nurses signed in.

The thirty-five-bed wards had a bright side, though. Having that many people in one room made it feel like a family where everyone helped everyone else. This was a blessing for poor people who might not have a family of their own. It was also a blessing for young trainees like me who were hesitant to get to know their patients but wanted to do the very best for them.

Despite the less-than-glamorous conditions, doctors had been eager to train at Bellevue for centuries because they would be exposed to the most distinguished professors, see every kind of medical diagnosis, and have the opportunity to solve difficult problems. One might hear of bed sores, but at Bellevue, one could see the very worst in ulcerated wounds.

I remember one man admitted to surgery to have his leg amputated. He had the largest leg wound anyone on the ward had seen. Even students from other services came to stand around his bed with those of us from Cornell to look in awe at his terrible wound.

It was clear to me his wound was not healing because his dressings were filthy every time his bandage was changed. So, I decided to increase the number of dressing changes to keep the wound clean at all times. As far as I could tell, this was not standard practice, but it saved the man's leg. Gradually, one could see evidence of healing at the edges of the wound, and the leg would survive. Later, I learned it was standard practice to use amputation instead of wound care with poor patients because it was less time-consuming.

Around this same time, the chairman of surgery called me into his office at New York Hospital. He told me that, as a woman, I had no business being in medical school. I was too pretty and would never actually practice medicine. I was taking the place of a man who could be there.

The male student I had replaced at Cornell eventually returned to school, so the chairman was wrong there, but his lecture and the treatment I received from him were humiliating. He refused to give me an externship at the hospital even though all the male students in my class were allowed to take one. My mentor at Bellevue gave me the news.

This was my first real rejection as a woman in medical school, and I wept. As such a privileged person in life, it had never occurred to me that bigotry could be directed at me. I had not yet learned that discrimination always has more to do with the psyche of the person discriminating than the person being discriminated against. I had yet to learn the real cost of discrimination to the person being targeted. I would get that later as a woman.

Despite this snub, the surgery department at Bellevue gave me an official citation for saving my patient's leg and an 'A' in the Surgery course. At the time, I even wondered whether the surgery chairman had rejected me because he was afraid I might pursue a career in surgery.

In 1965, President Lyndon Johnson pushed for the passage of Medicare for the elderly and Medicaid for the poor of any age as part of his Great Society legislation. This changed the world of medicine for hospitals like Bellevue. Now, the poor could go to wealthier hospitals, where they were welcomed with open arms—at least, welcomed until the advent of the AIDS epidemic.

My Pickpocket Patient

THE FIRST DAY I arrived at Bellevue, I was told the police were bringing in a patient for surgery who was on his way to jail for being a pickpocket and drug addict. I had never met someone like that before. I assumed pickpockets and drug addicts were depraved individuals to be avoided at all costs. I had already learned that even violent patients calmed down once the police left. But I was a little apprehensive meeting this new patient: a black man with a criminal record.

The resident doctor examined the patient and set him up for surgery. As a student, I was there to take a general history and make a record. I had never been this close to a black man before, but he was now my patient, so I needed to reach him. So, using my best social manner, I asked him, "Tell me, how do you pick someone's pocket?"

"If you stand a little closer, I'll show you," he laughed while explaining. "We only go after wallets because we haven't time to search your bag. The best way is to get someone known to the police to walk across 42nd Street, say. While the police watch that person, we grab all the easily exposed wallets." He also told me about his drug problem and his difficulty getting enough money to support his habit.

One day, shortly after this conversation, I was riding the elevator to my floor with one of my classmates and spotted a bandage cart from one of the other floors. On our floor, we were always short of bandages, so I got my fellow student to distract the man with the bandage cart while I stuffed my pockets.

When I got to the ward, I proudly told my pickpocket patient what I had done. To my great surprise, he was horrified. He took me aside and lectured me, "This is wrong. You must not take others' supplies. It will get you into a lot of trouble."

I did not think anyone was going to take me to task for pilfering bandages for my patients. Still, his concern for me and for having corrupted me moved my heart. In my mind, this man was supposed to be on the lowest rung of society, but here before me was a complex, caring human being who did what he had to do to survive. He picked pockets not because he thought it was right but because he felt he had to. But he did not want to hurt his young doctor, who had a promising future ahead of her.

One day, he asked to see me in the one private room on the floor. There, he thanked me for taking care of him. After that, he was gone, eloping from the hospital before he could be taken to jail.

This man's concern for me ensured that I would never forget

him, even after all these years. Knowing him meant I could never look at a black man, a drug addict, or any kind of so-called crook with the same judgmental eye I might otherwise have had.

Years later, in the 1990s, when I worked at the county hospital in Alabama, I saw once more how even the most honorable people at the bottom of society just don't play by the same rules we do in my world; they do whatever they must do to survive.

In Birmingham, patients sold their opiate medications just to have enough money to eat, keep a roof over their heads, or care for their children. I marveled at their lack of shame over going to jail or having a family member in jail.

Of course, in those days, I still thought convict labor was the useful work prisoners were assigned so they would have job skills when they got out of prison. I did not realize it was a kind of forced slavery, arresting the unemployed, then, because they did not have the money to post bail, sending them off to the coal mines or other chain gangs where they were brutalized and frequently died. I was still so innocent, I had no concept of the brutality and violence used in our criminal justice system against blacks, even up to the present. And how that brutality spilled over into medical treatment as well.

With my graduation from Cornell in 1964, I headed to Alabama for a medical internship with Dr. Tinsley Harrison of medical text-book fame. After one year in the South, I planned to take off for Boston and my residency in psychiatry at Mass General at Harvard.

I never imagined I would marry and stay in Alabama instead. I was a babe in the world of medicine, a babe in the world of race relations, and I was also a babe about the expectations of women in society, even marriage, especially in the South.

"*There is no fire like passion, there is no shark like hatred, there is no snare like folly, there is no torrent like greed.*"
— Buddha

"*Modern medicine is a negation of health. It isn't organized to serve human health, but only itself, as an institution. It makes more people sick than it heals.*"
— Ivan Illich

CHAPTER THREE

Lessons From the South

Moving to Alabama for an internship with Tinsley Harrison and then going to Harvard for my psychiatry residency seemed like a grand adventure. In Birmingham, I would be stepping into another world; I would be a doctor for the first time.

Arrangements had been made for me to live with my great aunt, Miss Belle, who had always been a source of strength and fun for the family. And I had lots of relatives and family friends in Birmingham to meet.

It was 1964 when I came to Birmingham, and the Civil Rights Movement dominated the news. The University Hospital was about to be integrated, and I heard a lot of angry racist talk. The year before, in Birmingham, peaceful demonstrations against Jim Crow had turned violent when the police got involved.

Then, in September 1963, members of the KKK bombed the 16th Street Baptist Church, killing four little girls. The police used dogs and fire hoses against demonstrators, most of them young African Americans. These developments shocked the nation and finally led to the passage of the Civil Rights Act of 1964, prohibiting discrimination on the basis of race, color, sex, and national origin in public accommodations. This officially ended Jim Crow in the South, but not the sentiments that had led to centuries of systemic mistreatment of blacks.

Coming from New York, I was prepared to support the cause of oppressed blacks, but I noticed when I attended meetings, the only white people there were Jewish. None of my family or the daughters of my mother's friends were there. I felt like I was living two lives.

Still, I Was Blind

MOVING TO THE SOUTH was more of a culture shock than I had expected, and the shock had as much to do with football as it did with integration and race relations.

EVERY WEEK, FROM WEDNESDAY to Friday, all the interns and residents at the hospital talked about who the University of Alabama football team would play the next Saturday. Then they talked about the previous week's game from Saturday to Wednesday. I'd been to school with a group of men, but had never heard anything like this football talk. It was obsessive. As University Hospital was being racially integrated, I heard a lot of negative talk about that, too, but football dominated the scene.

Afraid I might ride a bus, my parents gave me their second car. After that, I drove to work every day. I was one of only two women in the internship program. Everyone was very polite (especially compared to New Yorkers), so at first, I was not aware of how being a woman made a difference for me professionally.

However, I soon became conscious of being different, particularly when I sat with the other doctors as they talked about football. Still, I tried very hard to look the part of a doctor, proudly wearing my little white skirt and white jacket, the uniform that identified me as an intern or first-year doctor.

My Introduction to Healthcare Discrimination Against Blacks

My first rotation as an intern in July 1964 was in the Old Hillman Emergency Room. There, I was introduced to one aspect of black culture. On Friday nights, the emergency room was crowded with what the staff called "the gladiators."

Apparently, after work on Fridays, paycheck in hand, young black men headed to the bars to drink and fight. During that first month on call every other night, I saw a lot of knife and gunshot wounds. Surgery was on speed dial.

During my second month, I was transferred to the Veterans Health Administration (VA) Hospital. On my first night on the ward, I was up all night caring for a patient, a black man, who was admitted with difficulty breathing. The resident doctor in charge said he needed a tracheotomy, but not to bother because he was going to die anyway.

I had never done a trach on a human—only on a dog—but the medical student assigned to me had done one on a human, so while the resident sat in his office, the two of us did the procedure. When the patient died a few days later, I was forced to wonder, did this man die because we were too inexperienced or too aggressive during the tracheotomy? Or was he sent to us rather than surgery because he was black? Or had the resident simply been right from the start, and the man was going to die anyway?

Looking back, if the man was as sick as the resident suggested, should not the surgeons have done the tracheotomy and sent the patient to the ICU instead of sending him to me? At the time, my conscience was clear that I had done everything I could for my poor patient, but I was moved by his plight and profoundly confused.

Tuskegee Institute was not far away. Tuskegee was the site of a forty-year study on black men with syphilis. I was not aware of the history then, but I was horrified to learn later that the long-term study, which was conducted by the National Public Health Service and the Center for Disease Control (CDC) in collaboration with Tuskegee Institute, involved observing 400 rural black men with syphilis without offering treatment, even though treatment with penicillin had been readily available since 1947. The study did not end until 1972.

I was very formal with my patients back then, calling them all by their last names. I noticed how important it was to all my patients, but especially my black patients, to feel respected by me. Too often, other doctors spoke to black patients in a demeaning, discourteous tone, calling them "Boy" or "You."

I saw the disrespect toward black people and heard stories about how backward negroes were supposed to be, but I had no sense of the depravity of the Southern mistreatment of African Americans in medicine, education, and criminal justice. Somehow, naively, I thought the Civil Rights Movement was about separate bathrooms and water fountains, bus seats, and restaurant access. I knew nothing about medical neglect and experimentation, false arrests, convict labor,[4] and lynching. I had no concept of the depths to which many white people had gone to keep blacks terrorized so they would not vote and would stay disadvantaged in every way.

Meanwhile, I was focused on my own survival—how was I going to make it through the internship if I never got a good night's sleep again? So, I worked out a solution.

From then on, after morning rounds with all the patients and the attending physician, I headed for the on-call rooms and slept

4   The arrest of unemployed blacks who could not pay their bail, who were sent to work in the coal mines or some other chain gang where they were brutalized and often died.

until two in the afternoon. Then, I was back on the ward. I napped again from five to seven p.m. and then had the evening to see my patients, finish my charts, and deal with any problems.

I never had another all-night shift, but I was the best-rested intern all year. Taking naps also proved to be an efficient way to avoid drug reps and others who took up time during the day.

Meanwhile, I was growing as a physician, including learning some of the bureaucratic work I had to master. All too often, seeing patients involved in getting through the routine of the standard work-up, write-up, daily rounds, and orders, plus discharge planning, and the actual discharge process.

I learned from painful experience to get the chief resident to sign off on my discharges several days before I was ready to let patients go to avoid lengthy delays when the patient was, in fact, ready to go home.

Furthermore, when I was working at the VA, I learned that if I could evaluate and treat a patient in four hours or less, I did not even have to admit him to the hospital. Since so much of the hospital time was just waiting for test results or waiting for someone to check the patient, I figured out how to maximize those four hours for the patient's benefit and mine. That way, I could also keep my patient load to a minimum.

One day, I was told that a patient I had discharged the week before was being readmitted. Apparently, he had stopped taking his medicine and had become sick again.

When I walked into my patient's room, I was prepared to lecture him about the need to keep up with his medications. However, the look on his face made me pause. Here was this tall, gaunt black man dressed in hospital garb yet smiling from ear to ear. He held out a collection of pencils, notepaper, and peppermints in his large, bony hands. The patient wanted me to come look. The hospital volunteers had just left his room, and I assumed he was holding something they had given him.

With a tremor in his voice and tears on his cheeks, he showed me his treasures. "Now, I have something to give my grandkids for Christmas!" he said with a mile. Smart as I was supposed to be, it had never occurred to me that he might not take his medications because he could not afford them.

This man was a veteran. He looked like an old man to me, but he had young grandchildren, so he might not have been all that old. For the first time, I was able to see him as a human being with struggles beyond staying out of the hospital. This time, I was able to get social services to work on his problems before I discharged him again.

My Favorite Rotation

THE HIGHLIGHT OF MY year as an intern at University Hospital was my assignment to Dr. Abraham Russakoff. Dr. Russakoff was the ideal physician. He was highly trained and never saw his patients as cases or diagnoses. He knew their names, their families, and their life struggles.

I remember one night, a code was called for one of his patients who was dying. The patient had stopped breathing, and his medical team was trying to resuscitate him. As I stood with other interns watching the procedure to revive him, Dr. Russakoff told us about this patient and his life—what he had endured and what he had accomplished.

We were all impressed with the respect and care Dr. Russakoff showed to everyone in his care. Patients were not just numbers to be worked up and charted. While I seemed to spend most of my time as an intern just going through the routine, I admired his way of approaching patients.

My internship year went by quickly, with an engagement and wedding at the end. That fall, I met the man I was going to marry. I had planned to pursue a career in academic psychiatry, but there was no training program in psychiatry to be had in Birmingham, and it never occurred to me to ask my husband to accompany me to Boston so I could complete my training in psychiatry at Harvard.

Adventures in Research

IN THE MID-1960S, COMPUTERS were very new and not in general use in medical institutions. As a math major from Stanford, I knew more about computers than all the physicians I worked with, and more about medicine than those at the computer science center. Still, I was a real novice at both.

With great enthusiasm, I developed an elaborate statistical program using the data from the Cardiovascular Research Center. However, I was in for a shock. When I started to run the program, it was obvious the data I was feeding it was "garbage," a computer term meaning that something was seriously wrong with the data.

Checking the data, I realized you could not even compare two records taken on the same patient, on the same machine, on the same day, because the machine was not calibrated correctly. I also discovered that the person digitizing the records didn't reliably identify the onset of the electrical discharge on the electrocardiogram, the QRS complex, so any comparisons would not be using the same phase of heart contraction. Quite a few papers had been published using this data without anyone realizing the errors.

This was a huge lesson for me: Check everything for yourself!

Frustrated at the glitch in my planned research, I was glad to be leaving Alabama. I was now a married woman, and my husband and I were moving to Charlottesville, Virginia, where my husband would be in training to be a neurologist at the University of Virginia.

This was the 1960s. Long before the days of "Women's Liberation." I had been brought up to see marriage and raising a family as my main goals in life. My career in medicine was just the adventure I had until my real life: marriage and family began. After all, I was brought up being told, "Don't let the boys see how smart you are!" But being a doctor, when I married a doctor, meant I could not hide all of who I was.

Today making choices to follow your husband rather than pursue your own interests might seem old-fashioned, but today there are still many families, often heavily involved in the white Christian church, usually Roman Catholic or Evangelical Protestant, who preach that women should be subordinate to their husbands and need to follow their lead rather than their own interests. While other families encourage girls as well as boys to pursue education.

Looking back, I can see my family was somewhere in the middle. I'm sure if I had married young, I would have been happy in marriage and would have contributed through volunteer work, but I was already a physician in the middle of my training, and that was a problem.

Charlottesville

IN PLANNING OUR FUTURE, my husband and I did not look for a place where I could train in psychiatry while he trained in neurology. Instead, he planned to do his Neurology training in Charlottesville, so I found a research fellowship at the Virginia Heart Lab to use my experience with computers.

I was still imagining research in my future career. The Virginia Heart lab used a machine called a plethysmograph to measure changes in the blood vessels. They were interested in me because they were eager to purchase a computer and thought I might be of some help with their grant application.

On my first day, I was assigned to a lab and given a medical student to work with me. "Don't accept anything you are given without checking it for yourself," I cautioned, telling him about my experience in Birmingham.

The next day, he called me over. "This machine is not correct," he said. "It's producing twice as much pressure as it says it does." He pointed to the double column of water.

The thought of not accepting the machine's accuracy never crossed my mind because I was not good with mechanical things. Yet here was a device used in all the published studies coming out of this lab, and it was faulty.

Further checking showed that in some studies from the lab, they had used middle-aged men as controls for pregnant women. We arrived at very different results when we corrected the errors and repeated these published studies.

"What's in print is all that matters," My boss in the lab told me when we brought our results to him. "The head of this lab gets the most money out of the state legislature, so he can do no wrong at this institution." My experience at the Virginia Heart lab diminished my enthusiasm for research.

Then I learned I was pregnant. I decided to stop working for a while after I finished the year. However, the head of the lab pleaded with me to stay on for another year after the baby came, saying I could bring the baby with me to the lab.

My daughter, Anne, was the perfect baby for such a plan. She slept most of the day, only waking to be nursed every few hours. The arrangement was ideal, so I kept working.

"Only in the darkness can you see the stars."
— MARTIN LUTHER KING

"If some longing goes unmet we call that Life."
— ANNA FREUD

"What I have always wanted for myself is much more
primitive. It is probably nothing more than the
affection of the people with whom I am in
contact, and their good opinion of me."
— ANNA FREUD

CHAPTER FOUR

A Dark Period: Multiple Sclerosis, Divorce, and Male Bullying

During my time in Charlottesville, Virginia, I had my first symptom of multiple sclerosis, a dreaded disease that primarily starts in youth. My husband was training to become a neurologist. We had a tiny garage apartment out in the country overlooking the hills, half an hour west of Charlottesville.

I had just celebrated my thirtieth birthday when I realized I was pregnant. It was January, and the snow made a wonderland of the trees and mountains. My world seemed perfect. Then, one morning, I bent my neck forward and felt tingling all down my legs.

"What does that mean?" I asked my husband, the neurology resident, as he was getting ready to drive into the hospital for the day. I described what I was experiencing.

He looked horrified and said, "I hope you don't have that! It's Lhermitte's sign. It means you have multiple sclerosis!"

"Oh! I don't have that," I assured him, though I was careful not to bend my neck again. Every now and again, I thought about the tingling down my legs, but I did not bend my neck to test it again for months. When I did, the tingling was no longer there.

Before we left Charlottesville to return to Birmingham, I was pregnant again. Our son, Rob, was born the next February in Birmingham. Six months after that, I had an episode of numbness in my left leg.

The neurologist did a lumbar puncture (needle in my spine to get fluid) to check for elevated protein, common in multiple sclerosis, but it showed nothing. No one mentioned MS, and the doctor assured me that many people have small, minor neurological symptoms. This episode of numbness lasted about six months.

Back then, there was no MRI or definitive way of diagnosing MS. When the symptoms recurred two years later, I went to see a multiple sclerosis specialist at the university. He did not mention MS, and I was too scared to bring it up.

However, his words are seared into my memory: "This looks ominous." There was no internet to look up my symptoms, no one to share my fears with.

My relationship with my husband grew tense during this time, and we eventually divorced.

Entering the World of Biomedical Psychiatry

WHEN I FIRST STARTED my research fellowship in Birmingham, there were only seven neuropsychiatrists in the whole state of Alabama. However, in 1969, during my time in Virginia, the medical school in Birmingham added a Department of Psychiatry, where I was able to negotiate a special residency of training in psychiatry, taking four years instead of three. That way, I could spend more time with my children while they were small.

From the perspective of the early 1970s, psychiatry had already come a long way. The Roman Catholic Church dominated medicine and psychiatry in the Middle Ages. Individuals with severe mental illnesses were considered possessed by the devil. Thousands were burned at the stake.

We now realize that wildly crazy or demented individuals in the Middle Ages probably suffered from mania, severe depression, schizophrenia, or an array of unrecognized medical conditions, including seizures, infections like neurosyphilis, vitamin deficiencies, thyroid disease, and brain tumors. Those not burned at the stake as being in league with the devil were kept in asylums, chained up, neglected, and mistreated.

By the 19th century, psychiatry had become more humane. The great advance of that century was getting the mentally ill out of restraints and jails and into sanitariums, where they were given "moral therapy." This approach involved having a regular schedule, eating healthy food, and being productive at work. This approach helped many.

During the first part of the 20th century, the neurologist Sigmund Freud dominated psychiatry by uncovering the unconscious and developing a type of therapy called psychoanalysis, designed to address unconscious conflicts. Though human awareness of the unconscious had been known for centuries, Freud brought that awareness into the medical field, emphasizing the importance of the unconscious defense mechanisms[5] on all health and behavior, though influenced by the biases of the time, including misogyny.

Medical treatment of psychiatric disorders also advanced in this period, especially understanding conditions caused by vitamin deficiencies and infections like syphilis, which could be treated by penicillin beginning in the 1940s.

But it was not until the second half of the 20th century that

---

5   Unconscious mechanisms that distort realty to help us survive.

psychiatry was truly revolutionized by the discovery of medications to address psychosis and depression.

These medications—specifically, the mood stabilizer Lithium (1946), the antidepressant Imipramine (1951), and the antipsychotic Chlorpromazine (1952)—significantly improved the lives of institutionalized psychotic patients. Many were finally able to return to the community. Medication success led to a weakening of the psychoanalytic movement and the start of so-called Biomedical Psychiatry. This shift in psychiatry focused on finding the chemical imbalances in every human condition rather than studying the unconscious forces that drive so much of our behavior.

Biomedical psychiatry calls for the use of medications aimed at altering the disordered chemistry in the brain rather than addressing traumas, conflicts, or behavior through other forms of therapy or even addressing the nutritional aspects of the chemistry involved.

The psychiatry training program I attended in Birmingham was based on this biomedical approach. At the time, psychiatrists in biomedical training programs already were no longer required to have personal psychotherapy to understand their own conscious and unconscious issues that might interfere with their ability to treat patients. We certainly were not required to study any form of psychology or psychodynamics, which involves understanding the relationship between conscious and unconscious forces that affect our emotions and behavior and determine our personalities and motivation.

These subjects were not included in the bio-medical training program I attended in Birmingham to become a psychiatrist. I had to get that training on my own.

Beginning Training in Psychiatry

Starting my residency was often challenging. It had been four years since my medical internship when I had done physicals on patients. Sometimes, it felt like I had never had any medical training at all.

While doing my first physical exam, I got to the eyes and thought, "I have no idea what I'm looking for!" I was grateful for the knowledgeable nurses I could consult if I had any concerns.

Looking back, I can see I was much too concerned about myself. While seeing patients in the ER, I didn't want to look foolish by admitting someone to the hospital unnecessarily.

A case in point occurred during a recording of a patient interview intended for a teaching conference. While the tape was rolling during the interview, the patient leaned over and tried to kiss me.

I was so focused on not losing my cool that I failed to focus on what was going on with the patient and getting him to explore what his behavior meant. The incident on tape did make for a good lesson for my class presentation: stay focused on the patient and what the patient's words and behavior tell you about him.

It took me a while to focus completely on the patients rather than try to cover my own uncertainty. This lesson is vital if physicians are going to help patients and not just address their own concerns.

In the hospital, the attending psychiatrist initiated morning rounds in a group. All the patients gathered in one room, with the staff sitting in a circle. Everyone took a turn to talk and respond to others, allowing us to see all the patients at once and observe how they interacted with others.

The group setting also gave me a chance to watch the attending doctor in action, along with the nurses and the other psychiatric resident assigned to the ward. Group rounds were also helpful for medical students rotating through our service.

The group setting proved to be an effective way to help patients deal with their problems, and it was also a real godsend to me. It was my first lesson on the importance of getting suffering people to interact with others rather than go through their difficulties alone.

Instead of the know-it-all doctor dictating to the patient, wisdom came from all quarters. It was a lesson that served me well in working with patients throughout my career in medicine.

Having always been a good student, I soon mastered the routine. Since I started early in the morning and went home at noon per the terms of my four-year residency, the other resident doctor was left to handle the ward all by himself for the rest of the day.

One day, one of the nurses said to me, "You get more done in your time here than two of the other [male] residents."

I was certainly more motivated to get things done efficiently so I could leave early. But even though I worked hard to do my share of the work, from time to time, I sensed resentment on the part of the three-year-old residents, especially the other resident on my ward. I didn't fully understand the resentment, assuming it had to do with my getting off early. I didn't connect it to my being a woman at the time. My divorce was final by then, and I was adjusting to life alone with two young children to care for.

Six months into my residency, I was required to take part in a sensitivity training group. This sensitivity training group was to be our only therapy experience, and it was meant to teach us something about ourselves. The group was supposed to substitute for individual psychotherapy and was intended to help us understand our own internal dynamics. One of the local psychiatrists, Clause Hogland, was heading up the group.

I was really looking forward to the experience. I even thought it was kind of cool to be the lone woman in the group. I liked men and liked being around them. And while I had been discriminated against as a woman in medical school, I had no concept of what actual abuse could look like—that is, until I was attacked in the sensitivity training group.

Week after week, the men in the group talked about football and nothing else. I just watched and waited. The constant football talk in every session was one of the biggest culture shocks I'd experienced since coming to Alabama.

One day, as this group of future psychiatrists started up about football, I finally asked what our purpose was supposed to be in coming to the group. Suddenly, I was being hammered and trashed by each man in the group. Most of it is a blur. All I can remember is the large square table surrounded by men, all shouting at me.

I remember the resident I worked with saying, "I understand why you had to get a divorce!" And I remember Dr. Hogland saying, "There's something sticky or clingy about you." Everything else just felt like a steamroller had taken my breath and crushed me as a person.

For three days after that, I threw up every time I thought about what had happened. When I returned to work, I found I could not say a word except to my patients. I was mute with other people, even when I wanted to speak. Maybe I was too afraid I would burst into tears.

For some reason, I could not blame the group; I could only think about how loathsome I must be. I stopped going to church and even stopped calling my friends. It was all I could do to get through the day.

I had known I was experiencing discrimination in medical school when the chairman of surgery had said, "You're taking a man's place!" But I also knew I benefited in many ways from being a woman.

In addition to my scholarship, some professors let me do more than the men. And some looked out for me, even giving me special opportunities. This rejection by a group of Southern male psychiatrists was different, and I reacted with my whole being. I had no idea it had precipitated a major depression. I also had no idea this would be called male bullying.

When I returned to the group the next week, the man sitting beside me said he did not expect me to return. I did not say a word, and no one talked about what had happened the week before.

The following week, a new woman resident joined the group. She was a middle-aged woman who had been a pathologist. Dr. Hogland had been in medical school with this woman but had not seen her since. After the introductions, Dr. Hogland proceeded to take this woman apart by himself, much as I had been treated the week before.

It was shocking to watch, but no one spoke up. The next day, this woman committed suicide. I never knew the specifics of her life or why she was coming to train in psychiatry in her middle years. We were all stunned, but nobody talked about what had happened.

In the days after the suicide, no one in the department tried to process what had happened to us. No one tried to help the residents work through the suicide or what we had experienced in the group. Silence reigned. But the group never met again.

That experience should have been a lesson to me on the harm done by psychiatrists and other mental health professionals if they aren't forced to work out their own issues before they are unleashed on students or an unsuspecting public.

But in spite of seeing the viciousness of another woman being pummeled in the very same way I had been attacked, I was still too devastated by the group's assault on me just to throw it off. Even though the group ceased to meet after that, I was still traumatized. Without a meaningful effort to process traumatic events, those events can damage us internally, as they did me.

Fortunately, I did seek help when I was not better after a few weeks.

I had the great good fortune to be assigned to Dr. Clark Chase, a Freudian analyst who had retired to Alabama after twenty-five years of running the psychotherapy training program at the Menninger Clinic in Topeka, Kansas. Dr. Chase made a great point of showing me how psychiatrists with serious pathology themselves had still become influential in the profession.

Although it was not required as part of my residency training, I did seven years of twice-weekly psychotherapy with Dr. Chase and took part in weekly psychotherapy training as well. I also worked with a Jungian analyst, Janet Coltins, for seven years after that and spent a number of years doing group therapy with Joe Abbott, a family therapist and pastoral counselor, who rounded out my training.

It was interesting to see how psychiatry, like medicine itself, tended to focus on pathology, while the Jungian approach focused on signs of growth and positivity. By focusing only on the negative, whether it's a medical diagnosis or a personal loss, it's harder to encourage positive steps that will benefit the health of the patient.

Depression

IN THE DAYS FOLLOWING the group assault, I continued to attend lectures as part of my training program. In one session, the instructor brought up the subject of depression and listed its symptoms on the board.[6]

How can those be symptoms of depression? I thought. I have all those symptoms myself. I'm even losing weight without trying for the first time in my life.

I did indeed have symptoms of major depression, the first of two times in my life. I did not understand then that having a hopeless or helpless outlook on life is the most common symptom of depression, along with feelings of worthlessness, self-hate, or inappropriate guilt.

I remember I would wake in the night, unable to sleep, assailed by thoughts of how dreadful I was. In particular, I remember having some sherry one night to help me sleep and noticing how the thoughts were still there but no longer felt painful.

Not long after that, I was interviewing a woman who had become an alcoholic. I asked her, "How did you start drinking?"

"In my thirties, I started drinking sherry when I could not sleep at night. It progressed from there."

Horrified, I stopped having sherry right away.

Unfortunately, my doctor believed anti-depressant medication was not needed to treat my symptoms of depression since it was precipitated by a traumatic event. At the time, doctors assumed medication should be reserved for those with depression that emerges without an external trigger. We now know that antidepressant medications can help with symptoms of depression even if there are

6   Symptoms of depression: insomnia or sleeping too much, reduced appetite and weight loss or increased cravings for food and weight gain, loss of interest or pleasure in normal activities, feeling sadness, hopelessness, early morning fatigue, lack of energy for even small tasks, anxiety, agitation, or restlessness, feelings of worthlessness or guilt. Additionally, trouble concentrating or making decisions, thoughts of death or suicide, physical problems like back pain or headaches.

external triggers, originating from chronic illnesses like multiple sclerosis or chronic pain, or following PTSD after a traumatic event.

We also understand that processing the traumas from life with individual or group therapy is an important part of treatment, whatever the underlying cause of the depression. Having treated many patients in large groups, I wonder if group therapy is not more beneficial than one-on-one therapy, where you can reserve your secrets to yourself and not really expose them to the light of day.

Although I felt like crying every day after the group attack, I only cried once: the day a very sick boy with schizophrenia took me aside as he was leaving the hospital. "Thank you for treating me like a human being," he said.

I could see the suffering in his eyes. I wept openly. Looking back, I wonder if my own suffering made me more empathetic with the patients I saw in the hospital.

After the trauma I experienced in the group, all I could manage was work and taking care of my children. When I got better and returned to church, I did not feel the same way about the people I had known there. These people had been my best friends, yet I was hurt because they never called to see why I was not coming to church.

After I returned, I discovered they felt I had abandoned or rejected them. Since I still blamed myself for the group and was so ashamed, I did not share with anyone what had happened to me in the group, so there was no way they could understand why I had disappeared.

Furthermore, some of my women friends felt bitter because I had the advantage of having a degree, of being a doctor. These women I knew did not work, and some resented that I had a profession.

Behind my back, they called me a "queen bee." This was in an early phase of women's liberation. Locked in my depression, I did not realize that this meant to them someone who did not care about her sisters.

Undoubtedly, I withdrew from the support I might have had at church and with some of my women friends as a result of my depression. If I could do it over, I would like to think I wouldn't let myself withdraw like that; instead that I would reach out for help. But at the time, I was doing the best I could.

I learned later it's very British to keep things in, and having lived in England, I could certainly identify with being British. This was also true of my mother and grandmother, and may have been another factor in my withdrawal.

But being depressed filled me with a sense of shame. I blamed myself for being an awful person, which is common in depression. I also knew it wasn't safe to express my anger to my friends from church, the resident doctors who attacked me in the group, the group leader whose behavior had been so incredibly irresponsible, or the department head who failed to have the residents process what had happened to one of the residents or in the group. Instead, I had turned that anger against myself, which is also common in depression.

History of Attacks on Women Healers

EVEN THOUGH I WITNESSED a similar attack on another woman, I took the attack on me as being personal. Little did I know then that the source of violence has been directed at women in medicine, at least since the Middle Ages. I also did not recognize the attack on women healers as being part of medicine's attack on natural therapies, which I will discuss later.

"*I believe that you can, by taking some simple and inexpensive measures, lead a longer life and extend your years of well-being. My most important recommendation is that you take vitamins every day in optimum amounts to supplement the vitamins that you receive in your food.*"
— LINUS PAULING

Orthomolecular treatment does not lend itself to rapid drug-like control of symptoms, but patients get well to a degree not seen by tranquilizer therapists who believe orthomolecular therapists are prone to exaggeration. Those who've seen the results are astonished."
— ABRAM HOFFER, M.D., PH.D.

CHAPTER FIVE

Who Are the Charlatans? And What I Learned From Orthomolecular Psychiatry

Vacationing recently with my family on a barrier island, we were blessed with a house overlooking the tidal marshes of a bird sanctuary off the North Carolina Coast.

Every day as the tide ebbed and flowed, birds would fly in to fish or to probe in the mud for small creatures. To be one with nature was a treat for those of us slowed by the ravages of time. Half hidden by the fog on the marsh, the sun would rise slowly every morning, only to explode high in the sky at noon. Finally, as the sun retreated with the light of the day, we faced a canopy of multicolored splendor. We were part of that daily display of so much life and beauty.

Environmentalists had worked hard for many years to preserve the marsh at the end of the island for the birds. But every day at high tide, like a plague, a cohort of wave runners, their engines blaring, would race through the open channels of the marsh, ignoring those who lived there. They were followed by a cohort of men bringing nets to catch mullet by the bucket load.

The last remnants of land were being developed on the rest of the island. Indeed, loud machines reminded us daily that the beach and the island was now a mecca for too many people on vacation. The small bridge of the past is now replaced by a mega bridge with four lanes from the mainland. The island, once remote, is now crammed and overrun with people.

We Lose Our Connection to Nature in Medicine As Well

As I labored away on this book, I could not help seeing the connection between modern medical interventions and the tightly packed rows of rental houses on the barrier island we'd selected for our vacation. It was a modern explosion against the natural world, which is struggling to survive—the natural world we humans need to survive, too often treated as merely a setting for our convenience or pleasure.

How did it get this way? How did the Judeo-Christian traditions in the West see Nature just as something for humans to use, while most other religions, including Islam, have seen humans as part of that Nature— a Nature to be honored and supported? How do we fail to see our own link to nature? How has the practice of medicine carried us too far from the cures Nature affords us?

Few would look at the life-saving interventions of Western medicine and wish instead to be healed by a Shaman of old. Antibiotics and vaccines have had a miraculous effect on our survival. Many other treatments have meant a long life not to be had a century ago. And yet, with the best hi-tech medical interventions in the world, how does our health care in the U.S. rate so far behind other countries?

Yes, we rank number one in the world in medical technology, but we rank 97th in the world in the quality of our health care! Can it be that Western medicine embraces technology instead of the full range of what humans need to heal?

My first exposure to the problem occurred in 1975. As a senior resident in psychiatry, I was attending my first psychiatric meeting, the World Congress for Psychiatry in Honolulu, Hawaii.

After a fascinating week of listening to all the world's experts in psychiatry, I went to hear the Orthomolecular psychiatrists. During the meeting, I had heard the biomedical psychiatrists criticize the psychoanalytic psychiatrists and vice versa, but there was a special hostility toward this orthomolecular group. I remember being surprised at the amount of venom directed at these physicians.

Orthomolecular[7] Psychiatry

ALL I KNEW ABOUT these doctors at the time was what was being said about them by my professors back home: "These Orthomolecular doctors are frauds to claim vitamins are going to cure schizophrenia. They give massive doses of vitamins, and yet they also use anti-psychotic medicine just like we do. Anti-psychotic medication is what makes the difference!"

---

7   "Orthomolecular" is defined as "pertaining to a theory that illness can be treated and health maximized by creating the optimal molecular environment for the cells of the body through the introduction of natural substances." The concept about the importance of vitamins was introduced by Nobel Prize winner Dr. Linus Pauling in the late 1930s. In the mid-1960s, he became intrigued with the biochemistry of nutrition. Pauling began his research looking for causes of mental retardation and mental illness (especially schizophrenia.) He believed these conditions were caused by biochemical disorders in the brain. In founding the new field of orthomolecular psychiatry, Pauling proposed that mental abnormalities might be treated by correcting imbalances or deficiencies of naturally occurring substances in the brain, notably vitamins and other micronutrients, as an alternative to synthetic drugs. In 1968, Pauling broadened this concept into orthomolecular medicine, which is based on the physiological and enzymatic actions of specific nutrients, such as vitamins, minerals, and amino acids present in the body.

Saturday was the last day of the conference, and I still had not been to the beach. The only items on the program that day were talks by orthomolecular psychiatrists. My buddies planned to skip these sessions to go sightseeing. I studied the program, trying to decide how to spend my day. The orthomolecular psychiatrists at this meeting were presenting several papers on basic research, plus clinical studies of patients with schizophrenia.

Looking at the program, I suddenly decided I really wanted to see what "charlatans" looked like. I was unprepared for the shock I would get when I listened to what these doctors said, but I knew I had to attend the session. At the time, I had no idea I was witnessing an attack on natural therapies by regular medicine

Charlatans

I FOUND THE VERY small meeting room and slipped into my seat. As I retrieved my notebook, I noticed there were very few participants, unlike the groups gathering to hear the talks about medications, but many people there seemed to know one another.

When they started presenting papers, I was impressed to see these doctors were conducting careful scientific research on various aspects of schizophrenia and its treatment. I had trouble following many of the biochemical studies because I lacked the right scientific training. These orthomolecular psychiatrists were extremely knowledgeable physicians. Listening to their talks, I could see they were looking at all aspects of their patients' function and dysfunction.

In the hours that followed, I learned that they used anti-psychotic medications to treat their schizophrenic patients' psychosis, just like the rest of psychiatry. But they also used the latest discoveries in nutrition and medical care, as well as all advances in psychiatry to help their patients.

Paying attention to nutrients and their patients' physical condition meant their patients were healthier. Using individual and family therapies to work out individual and family problems helped their patients live more stable lives—no small feat for people with schizophrenia. Having stable lives meant their patients were able to take lower doses of anti-psychotic medication to control their psychotic symptoms. And lower medication doses meant they took their medicine because they had fewer side effects. As a result, these patients did well over a long period of time!

To my amazement, these despised physicians were the only psychiatrists I'd heard all week who acknowledged and used all of the advances in psychiatry, medicine, and nutrition to help their patients. They were not promoting vitamins as an alternative to anti-psychotic medication or problem-solving. They addressed all aspects of their patients' lives with what was available then. And these doctors were the charlatans?

The fact that they were using every kind of therapy out there to maximize their patients' health and well-being impressed me at the time. But it also made understanding other physicians' resistance to their approach harder. I was still naive enough to believe that all doctors were seeking the best and safest treatments for their patients—not just advancing their own careers or specialties and making compromises at their patients' expense, both knowingly and unknowingly.

I also failed to recognize how unconscious defenses would drive physicians to pursue professional directions that would benefit themselves, even if not all of their patients. And I failed to see how pursuing concrete solutions was in itself an unconscious defense against anxiety, much like Descartes' pursuing treatment of the body like a machine was a "Flight to Objectivity."[8]

The history of medicine is replete with groups of doctors doing the right thing but being discredited by other doctors who want control or power, not better medical care. In the 1840s, the Hungarian Dr. Ignaz Semmelweis was run out of town for suggesting doctors were inadvertently bringing something from the autopsy room into the birthing room that was making new mothers sick.

In reality, doctors were causing childbed fever by carrying germs on their hands. Midwives had fewer cases of infant and maternal mortality because they were not exposed to germs before delivering babies. Was this another example of professional blindness?

Perhaps, but this was also before Louis Pasteur's discovery of germs in 1861. And midwives were females in competition with men.

Although I observed this apparent professional blindness in 1976, I did not make the connection between the biomedical training program I was in and the attack on natural therapies. Nor did I recognize how biomedical psychiatry was focusing on the concrete by promoting medications over all other interventions.

I also did not recognize that failing to train psychiatrists in psychotherapy or insisting that they go through personal therapy themselves to understand their own issues would mean psychiatrists were more likely to inflict their own biases on their patients and students. I had even observed the cost of such neglect myself, but did not recognize it for what it was until later.

---

8   Susan R. Bordo, *The Flight to Objectivity: Essays on Cartesianism and Culture,* *1987.*

Skip to Today

IN THE MORE THAN fifty years since that meeting in Hawaii, the whole profession of psychiatry and most psychiatrists have embraced medications over all other forms of therapy. They have not done the hard work of having personal therapy to work out their own issues.

In fact, many psychiatrists today do not offer any forms of therapy other than medication in their offices, though they may have psychologists and social workers who do. But as a result of this limited focus and training, biomedical psychiatry has tried too hard to treat everything with medication rather than reach a more balanced approach to treatment.

Today, in the ultimate irony of ironies, among the seriously mentally ill that we psychiatrists are supposed to treat are many homeless people, leading unstable lives on the streets without access to psychiatric care except in emergencies. If they commit any acts of violence or even threaten violence, they may find themselves confined to prison for years.

Many of the homeless use street drugs and end up with psychosis, get hospitalized, are treated with high doses of anti-psychotic medication, and then are discharged again to the street. There, they stop taking their medication because they don't like the side effects and end up psychotic again: the revolving door.[9] They are even free to use their government SSI checks to buy the street drugs that make them crazier.

Looking back, I realize the orthomolecular psychiatrists had

9   Wyatt v Stickney in 1964 ruled that hospitals cannot hold the mentally ill against their will if they cannot offer treatment. This led to the emptying of mental hospitals and loss of facilities to house and treat the mentally ill across the nation. It vastly contributed to the homeless problem in this country.

it right when they focused on medical, nutritional, and individual and family therapy to ensure a healthy, stable environment while also prescribing anti-psychotic medications. A recent study from the National Institutes of Health (NIH) shows that schizophrenics do better with some psychotherapy.[10] What a surprise!

Unfortunately, psychiatry is still enthralled by the rest of medical practice. That is, it is based on the biomedical model's approach to patients. Some psychiatrists are now beginning to see the benefit of addressing all aspects of living, from treating the cellular cause of illness or behavior to dealing with psychological and relationship issues in the individual and the family to addressing things like community support and environmental issues. Even if that means leaving the psychosocial aspects of psychiatry to psychologists and social workers.

In 1976, I did not understand psychiatry's treatment of Linus Pauling and the orthomolecular group, but I was able to see firsthand how the medical profession tried to discredit those taking a different approach to treatment. Even though I kept seeing this disconnect between the best therapy and the attitude of my profession, I had no idea what the underlying dynamic was until much more recently.

10   Paul H. Lysaker, Ph.D.; Shirley M. Glynn, PhD; Sandra M. Wilkniss, PhD, and Steven M. Silverstein, PhD, "Psychotherapy and Recovery from Schizophrenia: A Review of Potential Applications and Need for Future Study," Psychol Serv, 2010, 7(2): 75-91.

"*The unfortunate thing about this world is that good habits are so much easier to give up than bad ones.*"
— Somerset Maugham

"*All the suffering, stress and addiction comes from not realizing you already are what you are looking for.*"
— Jon Kabat-Zinn

CHAPTER SIX

What Drugs and Addiction Taught Me

For my fourth year as a resident in psychiatry, I was asked to head up one of the three psychiatric treatment teams as a junior faculty member. I was told this assignment was in lieu of being chief resident in my final year of residency. The treatment teams had inpatient and outpatient responsibilities staffed by a psychiatrist, a psychologist, a social worker, and various nurses.

As it turned out, nearly all my team members were female. I was lucky. In the seventies, since many fields were not as open to women as they are today, many of the most talented women became social workers, nurses, and psychologists.

The only man on my treatment team was the exercise therapist. When I went to talk to him about what he was doing with the patients, he said no doctor had ever bothered talking with him before. By then, I was used to conducting staff business and patient rounds in a team setting and urged the exercise therapist to join.

As a team, we solved problems in the outpatient clinic as well as in the hospital. Getting patient system-wide charts delivered to the clinic was always a problem, so we decided to keep records of our own. That helped us individualize treatment plans and be more effective with patients.

In the department's end-of-year report, the chairman's secretary announced our treatment team had treated the most patients, had the fewest complaints, and made the most money. Our success should have been a good thing, but within a week, I noticed that members of my team were being transferred elsewhere. When I asked the chairman why they were dismantling the treatment team that had been so effective, the chairman told me he wanted physician-directed teams rather than having all team members be part of the decision-making process. He wanted a top-down management style rather than a collaborative one.

Then, he told me that for my first year on the faculty, he would be transferring me to the team treating drug abuse. The medical director of that team was leaving, and I would be taking his place until they found a replacement.

I knew nothing at all about drug abuse, but growing up in a Navy family, I was used to being thrown into new situations and having to adjust. So, I studied drugs, drug addiction, and the treatment of alcoholics and addicts. In the early 1970s, the Drug Abuse Treatment Program was funded by a federal grant set up to deal with the growing problem of addiction in the country. The Drug Abuse Team had been working together for several years when I took over.

History of Drug Use and Abuse in the United States

MIND-ALTERING DRUGS HAVE BEEN used for medicinal and recreational purposes in the United States since their inception. In 1890, the Sears, Roebuck, and Co. catalog even offered a syringe and a small amount of cocaine for $1.50. Some states attempted to regulate drugs and alcohol, but it was not until 1914, when Congress passed the Harrison Act, that the federal government tried to regulate and tax the production, importation, and distribution of opiates and cocaine. This regulatory fervor led many physicians to shy away from using opiates with their patients for many years.

In the 1970s, the federal government under Richard Nixon started the War on Drugs, especially focused on opiates and cocaine. It was also the beginning of federally funded treatment programs aimed at addicts.[11]

My Experience with Drug Abuse

INITIALLY, I COULD SEE that members of the Drug Abuse team were resentful of having a novice assigned to lead them. Many felt I not only did not know about drug abuse, but that I should have experienced addiction myself and become a recovering addict to be effective in treating addicts. I could sense the hostility and resistance to including me in treatment decisions. Still, I had some successes with patients and even learned about the use of opiates in the treatment of pain after surgery.

One patient, a nurse admitted to our unit for opiate addiction, needed to have emergency surgery after being in the program for several weeks. When she was first admitted, she made it clear she did not want to deal with me. The drug treatment team seemed delighted to abet her.

The doctor doing her surgery said she would need opiates after the operation to manage her pain. The drug team staff was adamant that she be transferred off our floor before the surgery because, under the terms of our government contract, we could not give opiates on the unit except for detox.

---

11   "War on Drugs," editors: History.com.

I went to see the patient to explain the situation. "I don't want you to suffer after the surgery," I told her. "But I also don't want to interfere with your treatment for opiate addiction by giving you opiates. You're doing so well in your treatment program, and we would have to transfer you off this unit to give you opiates for pain. If you want, I can work with you to determine what you need and see if we can avoid having to transfer you."

She was eager to try.

After the surgery, I went to see the patient several times through-out the day. I brought her magazines and hard candy. I arranged for staff and other patients to visit her and encourage her. As it turned out, she had an easy time and did not require opiates.

"Thank you for believing in me," she said when I went to see her the next day. "I didn't want to deal with you before because I was not sure I wanted to have treatment for addiction. I was being forced into this program with threats of losing my nursing license. I can hardly believe I did not need opiates after the surgery!"

This was an early lesson for me about the importance of the doctor-patient relationship in managing pain and other conditions without medication. It was also an early lesson in pain management. I learned that taking opiates is not the only way to deal with pain, even post-op.

Opiates can be lifesaving when given to patients after a heart attack or severe burns. Opiates may even facilitate recovery from surgery or injury by getting people up and moving around sooner. But opiates are not the only way to bring this about.

Too often, giving patients opiates initiates a dependence on pills to manage pain and promotes the addiction we see across this country. Sadly, just like opting for amputation rather than taking the time to do wound care, using opiates is a quicker way to get patients going than spending time with them.

At the end of my year as medical director of the drug abuse team, the pharmacology department asked me to lecture sophomore medical students about addiction in their pharmacology course. I decided to ask one of the addicts on the unit to join me and reveal his secrets to the students while I gave facts about addiction.

The students were transfixed while my patient told them how he tricked the docs in the emergency room into giving him drugs. As for me, I still had not fully recovered from the group attack I experienced in my first-year sensitivity group. I was so nervous I could hardly get my words out.

Still, the Pharmacology department liked my dog and pony show, so for the next thirteen years, even after I went into private practice, I was invited back to sophomore pharmacology to lecture about addiction.

After a few years, I added to lectures on the medical uses of drugs that tend to be abused: opiates for pain, sedatives for sleep, tranquilizers for anxiety, and stimulants for depression. During this period, naturally occurring opiates, the endorphins and enkephalins, were discovered, along with the opiate receptors in the brain that opiates fit like a key in a lock.

During those thirteen years, I taught in pharmacology, I also taught about Physician Impairment[12] in the Introduction to Medicine Course for Juniors. By then, I had realized that all humans have blind spots, and I spent many of my lectures with medical students explaining that the modern practice of medicine and medical education was only one way of addressing health, just not the only way.

12   Physician impairment is a euphemism for drug and alcohol problems, even though other conditions can cause physicians to become impaired.

During that period, I was providing the only education medical students got about addiction in medical school. Doctors believed addiction was not a problem in the medical profession or even for white people. Even though white people are as susceptible to addiction as minorities, drug use has been so effectively demonized by being associated with minority communities that the whole medical response to addiction has been to dismiss it.

In addition, as a whole, the medical profession was in denial about the presence of addiction within its own profession. Two things happened in the 1970s to change that. First, the profession had to investigate a rash of physician suicides in Oregon in the early 1970s. They found the state had initiated punitive regulations affecting physicians using drugs or alcohol, ruining many physicians with drug and or alcohol problems.

In addition, cocaine became a popular drug of abuse. It may take thirty years to become an alcoholic who can't hide his drinking, but cocaine use by doctors gets them into trouble quickly.

Suddenly, the medical profession was forced to recognize addiction as a professional hazard for doctors and other healthcare professionals. Access to drugs, as well as the high stress of the profession, contributed to this hazard.

Programs for treating physician addicts popped up in Georgia and Mississippi, but this did not change the stigma attached to being an addict. After my first year, I looked for a physician addict to talk with the students. The doctor who volunteered to speak to my class was a recovering alcoholic in his fifties. Even though he did not look seedy, I realized I saw him that way anyway. (The prejudices of the time ran deep.) Eventually, a treatment program in Mississippi sent groups of young doctors from their treatment program to talk with the students during my lectures. These young doctors got into trouble early after using cocaine. They were all white physicians.

Most doctors were so ignorant about addiction and pain management during this time that they avoided prescribing opiates for pain. They tended to be uneducated about how opiates work and how to use them most effectively. That meant they used too few opiates for their patients who could benefit, even when it was lifesaving, and even when opiates were needed to break the pain cycle to get people going again after surgery.

Unless someone was dying, which might mean any amount of opiate was all right, doctors were very leery about giving any opiates. Opiates fell into that category of subjects in medicine that tend to be most misunderstood: areas dealing with emotions. Among other things, doctors did not realize that opiates only treat the emotional aspects of pain. That is, they have no effect on nociception (the peripheral perception of discomfort) or the pain threshold. Like the sherry I drank in the middle of the night, that didn't change my thoughts but blunted the pain I felt over them, so opiates affect the suffering that accompanies pain, not the awareness of discomfort.

By the time I got into treating chronic pain in the 1990s, the whole approach to opiates had changed. By then, doctors were prescribing lots of opiates both after surgery and for chronic pain, reaching a peak consumption by 2012 when Americans were consuming 80% of the world's pain medications (opiates).

Doctors had shifted from giving no opiates to giving too many opiates, especially the very strong synthetic opiates like OxyContin. In the process, they were promoting more pain as well as addiction, completely neglecting the many natural ways to treat pain, especially chronic pain, some of which have been known for thousands of years, like distraction and shifting focus to one's deep breathing.

Once more, I was observing the lack of understanding about natural therapies, but I still had not discovered the root cause.

Sometimes, we forget that wear and tear, illness, or injury may result in a weakened area of the body that is going to hurt from time to time. In addition, both overdoing and inactivity may lead to muscle spasms, shortening of tendons, or other changes that bring discomfort or pain. Even pain from trapped nerves can be shifted by focused exercise and stretching.

Furthermore, depression and PTSD have chronic pain as one of their symptoms. If we see pain pills, especially daily opiates, as the only answer for pain, we have missed the chance to develop the habits that serve us well in managing depression and chronic pain that are inevitable for everyone at times throughout life.

"*As any doctor can tell you, the most crucial step toward healing is having the right diagnosis. If the disease is precisely identified, a good resolution is far more likely. Conversely, a bad diagnosis usually means a bad outcome, no matter how skilled the physician.*"
— ANDREW WEIL

"*There is only one cardinal rule: One must always listen to the patient.*"
— OLIVER SACKS

"*Never deny a diagnosis, but do deny the negative verdict that may go with it.*"
— NORMAN COUSINS

CHAPTER SEVEN

What MS Taught Me About Chronic Illness

In the spring of 1977, after nearly ten years of sensory symptoms that came and went, I was finally diagnosed with multiple sclerosis. That year, the American Psychiatric Association met in Atlanta. During the meeting, I became aware of having new symptoms.

First, I noticed I could not make myself step onto the escalator. As a psychiatrist, it seemed so strange that I assumed I had developed an escalator phobia, an irrational fear of escalators. I did remember I had been hiking with my children the week before and had felt afraid to climb down a steep hill. Maybe something else was going on.

During the meeting, I went to Underground Atlanta with some of my colleagues and their friends. Being the only female there, I got to dance all night. I was in heaven. When I woke up the next morning, though, I had a clumsy left leg and numbness and tingling in both legs.

This time, the neurologist admitted me to the hospital to run some tests. "You have multiple sclerosis!" the doctor announced triumphantly as he entered my room, smiling like the Cheshire Cat. He had my newest test, a CT scan, in his hand.

He proudly showed me the hole in my brain, which meant I had multiple sclerosis.

"You have a Brown-Séquard syndrome,[13] which means you have different effects on each side of your body."

In my case, I have weakness in the front of the left leg and in the back of the right leg. I have numbness on the left and heightened sensation on the right, and my right leg often feels painfully cold. I also experience changes in proprioception, or feeling where my foot is in space, which makes it hard to put my foot on a moving escalator because I cannot feel where I am putting my foot.

Looking at the hole in my brain as the doctor held up the scan, I was devastated. At this point, ten years after that first twinge down my legs, you would think I'd have already known I had multiple sclerosis. It certainly crossed my mind every time I had a new episode. And yet, being told I had multiple sclerosis while looking at the scan came as a shock.

I suppose I had been lying to myself, telling myself that having multiple sclerosis could not possibly be that bad. I had told myself it was just little sensory changes every few years that eventually went away. Even after a previous episode with loss of vision in my left eye (optic neuritis) had resolved so quickly, I told myself it was just a side effect of the flu shot. After all, lots of people had neurological symptoms after getting that particular vaccine. However, this official diagnosis of multiple sclerosis was different.

For the first time, I had symptoms of motor dysfunction, which affected my walking. Now, even worse, the CT scan revealed that I

---

13   Brown-Séquard syndrome is defined as having motor weakness on one side with loss of knowing where you are in space (proprioception), combined with a loss of pain sensation and temperature on the other side. It's caused by a lesion in the spinal cord, specifically in the neck or cervical area.

had a hole in my head. I supposed it was an enlarged ventricle, but I was too traumatized to get the specifics. As a doctor, I ran CT scans on all my patients with symptoms of Alzheimer's disease, and they were always normal. What was happening to my brain? The doctor didn't tell me what this hole meant or what to expect. No one told me anything, and I was too stunned to ask.

I had always been called a "brain." The one area in which I had complete confidence in myself was my brain, especially my judgment and ability to figure things out. And there was obvious damage to that organ. How would I ever be able to trust myself again? Was it even safe for me to see patients?

I felt devastated while this doctor just sat there looking pleased with himself for making the diagnosis. "What can I do?" I asked, desperate to have a plan to deal with my loss.

"There's nothing you can do," he said. "Just don't burn the candle at both ends.'"

What does "don't burn the candle at both ends" even mean? I have a medical practice. I'm raising two children on my own. I have an elderly mother who needs my help.

The doctor wanted me to return in three months, but since he had nothing to offer me and was making me feel worse, I decided to stay away. Every time I had a new symptom, I just assumed it was multiple sclerosis and looked for ways to handle it on my own.

Today, we know that both exercise and antidepressants can increase the size of the corpus callosum, the part of the brain connecting the right side with the left side. So that physical therapy might have been worth trying to regrow the hole in my brain. But of course, we did not have that information in 1977. We did not even know from the CT what exact area in my brain was affected. I stayed home with my children for a week after the diagnosis, hoping my clumsiness would go away, just like the loss of vision had in the past. This time it did not.

MS Affects My Life

WHEN I RETURNED TO work, I went to see the Chairman of Psychiatry to tell him about my multiple sclerosis diagnosis. Within days, he sent me an official termination letter giving me two weeks' notice. Apparently, the chairman did not know he could not fire me abruptly like this. As a faculty member, I had a year to make other arrangements before I left. Today, I might have had more protections, but this was a decade before the Americans with Disabilities Act was passed.

Thwarted in his attempt to get rid of me right away, the chairman went further; he pulled me out of my leadership role on the drug abuse team and sent me to the outpatient clinic to do physicals. I was hurt, but I was determined to give it my best.

I bought a stethoscope and held my head high as I went to the clinic to examine patients. But I soon realized that after the change, I was now a pariah in the department. Everyone became less friendly. I don't know who knew what, but I was clearly out of favor.

In addition to running the drug team the previous year, I was responsible for the resident teaching program. I also developed an educational program for psychiatrists around the state who needed to review material for specialty boards. Because different people prefer visual, auditory, or experiential ways of learning, I even provided various ways of absorbing the material.

I'd been responsible for hundreds of hours of coursework, but when I showed up at an education meeting, the chairman thanked everyone for their service—even those responsible for only six hours of coursework—but he never once mentioned me or thanked me.

Worst of all, he announced who would be in charge of resident teaching for the next year. I was stunned. How could anyone be so vile as to let me know I had been replaced in front of my peers without telling me in person first?

I had already heard the chairman disliked me before my diagnosis, since he had told my mentor that tall women repelled him. "She reminds me of an aunt I hated," he apparently had said. My mentor told me this because he didn't want me to be hurt by the chairman's behavior since his actions were based on his own biases, not on my performance or my illness. Unfortunately, this only added to my feelings of desperation about having a hole in my head.

Multiple Sclerosis Affects Other Relationships

TRAUMATIZED BY THESE EVENTS, I confided in the man I was dating about having multiple sclerosis and what was happening with my job. He did not stop dating me right away, but it was soon clear he was calling less often. I began telling myself that maybe he had problems with intimacy because his mother had had schizophrenia, and that might also explain the fact that he was in his thirties and had never been married.

Then, one day, I walked into a church meeting, and there he was with a younger woman. Even though he later married a different woman, I still cannot see that first woman without reliving the pain I felt at the moment. Once again, I was devastated.

This event even brought on another episode of major depression. I could not sleep at night, and I also lost weight without trying. After this rejection, I was afraid to tell anyone I had multiple sclerosis. I looked mostly normal, of course, and lots of people limp for various reasons, so the multiple sclerosis was essentially invisible to the world. Still, with a hole in my head, I wanted to be sure it was safe for me to see patients. As a precaution, I saw a psychiatrist and, later, a psychologist to be sure.

However, keeping my MS a secret also meant I was not sharing with friends. In retrospect, I could have gone to group meetings at the Multiple Sclerosis Society, but I was afraid no one would come to me as a patient if word got out about my condition. Plus, I was so depressed that I would burst into tears when I tried to talk about it. Looking back, I can see that isolating myself so much was a huge mistake. It meant I was no longer close to my friends.

In hindsight, it would have been helpful if the neurologist had given me activities I could master as a way of dealing with my illness. We all neglect ourselves in some way or another until an illness forces us to focus on healthy living. We have long understood that focusing on healthy living always gives us the best chance of recovering from any illness. This was true even then.

Although the science demonstrating the link between exercise and the size of various areas of the brain had not been done at that time, a focus on healthy living always gives the individual the best chance of recovery from anything. As a psychiatrist, it concerns me that the medical profession categorizes exercise and diet as "lifestyle changes" rather than as means to facilitate recovery. This means doctors can dismiss these areas as too peripheral and too time-consuming to discuss with their patients.

In my days of working with medical students, I always taught them how important it is for the doctor to give the patient something tangible to work on or focus on to improve. I wanted the students to understand there is always an element in the transaction between doctor and patient that makes the medicine more effective: something beyond the chemistry of the pill—something facilitating the healing process. Looking back, I suppose I was talking about what we call the placebo effect and the mysterious effect of the doctor-patient relationship on healing. Too many doctors have been ready to dismiss these powerful healing forces.

Now, in addition to the boost to healing offered by the placebo effect, I can see the importance of giving the patient something they can do themselves, something that gives them some control back over their own health and lives. It can be as simple as telling you to put ice on your injury, walk up and down the hall four times a day, drink lots of water, meditate, and focus on your breathing when you walk.

As a patient and psychiatrist, I have understood this: a doctor with nothing to give but bad news is not in a position to help the patient. In fact, negative expectations can actually make patients worse. Doctors need to provide focused targets for improvement rather than focus on the negative, especially when dealing with chronic illnesses.

Still, I was lucky, at least for a few years. The Dean of Medicine hired me to work with medical students and be his Affirmative Action Officer before I was returned to the Department of Psychiatry. I eventually left to go into private practice.

"Opportunities to find deeper powers within ourselves
come when life seems most challenging."
— JOSEPH CAMPBELL

CHAPTER EIGHT

What Injury Taught Me About Recovery from Pain

In my youth, I was drawn to sports. I played tennis and swam, rode horseback, and loved square dancing. I joined the rock-climbing club at Stanford and rappelled off the chemistry building. One year, I even climbed Cathedral Spire in Yosemite.

In medical school, I rode horses around New York's Central Park reservoir before class every morning, played squash with my classmates, and thought skiing was magical. How grand the physical strength of youth is and the faith one has in one's ability to do anything!

When I moved to Alabama, which has more navigable rivers than any other state in the continental US, I discovered canoeing and camping. It was such a treat to be outdoors and close to nature. But later, in my forties, when MS gave me a foot drop, I would often trip and fall, especially in the woods. On one outing, I tripped climbing into my canoe and landed hard on my backside. After that, I was in so much pain I could neither sit nor stand without agony.

Tests did not show any broken bones, but I was in too much pain even to walk for exercise. I saw various doctors, but they all just gave me a shot of cortisone and sent me to physical therapy (PT) for several weeks. PT would help for a while, but then, the pain and leg spasms returned with a vengeance. I was constantly having to get up and stretch just to be able to sleep at night.

Once, I loved going to the symphony, plays, and lectures, but I could no longer comfortably sit through the performances. When I went to see the musical Les Mis, though the performance enthralled me, I had to leave in the middle.

I grew increasingly depressed during this period and gained fifty pounds. I always eat too much when I'm down, especially when I'm not exercising. I felt like a beached whale.

Desperate to get my life back, I went to a weight loss clinic. In eight months, I shed the fifty pounds. I started with a powdered diet, but after a couple of months, I was able to shift to regular food and continue losing weight. My success gave me such a superior feeling. Having struggled with weight all my life, I felt I had finally found the answer.

When I went out for lunch with friends, they were eating boring diet food while I was having the most delicious morsels, just in very small quantities. What a fantasy, thinking I could keep eating tiny amounts and not start craving more! Now we know that many foods in the profit-driven American food market affect our brains, so we want to keep eating. After two months at my ideal weight, I noticed I was gaining. Horrors!

I had read somewhere that walking an hour a day could keep the weight off. So, even though I hurt with every step I took, I started walking up and down my upstairs hall: back and forth, back and forth. I thought, if I'm going to hurt anyway, I may as well walk.

At first, I had to stop and stretch every few feet to lessen the pain, but I could stretch enough to keep going. Gradually, I worked up to walking an hour a day. My pace was very slow since I had a limp, and every time the pain returned, I stopped and stretched my heel down on a step or put a leg up on the arm of a chair before I hobbled on some more.

After a few months of walking up and down my hall for an hour, I decided to move outside and walk up and down the alley behind my house. The alley was mostly flat, with a gradual slope at one end. The first day of venturing outside before dawn, I kept expecting someone to jump out at me. There was a streetlight nearby, so it was not completely dark as I climbed the stone stairs behind my house up to the alley above.

Once I reached the alley, I had to laugh at my nervousness—the whole neighborhood was out walking! They were not in my alley, but I could see them walking up the hill in front of my house, coming around the bend, and walking past the entrance to my alley to take the street behind my house. So, I plugged my headphones into my Walkman for music and started to walk back and forth, moving as fast as I could.

Still in pain, I had to stop and stretch every time I turned around. Sometimes, I stretched on the back steps, sometimes on the stone wall. I always took a pot of hot tea and a tea cozy with me up the steps so I could take a few sips of hot tea with each lap. To my relief, I could keep walking as long as I stretched, and even though the pain and leg spasms came back later in the day, walking did not make the pain worse. My weight stabilized and even came down a little. My spirits improved, too, and I began doing more things with friends.

Before walking, I had been accustomed to going from my air-conditioned or heated house to my air-conditioned or heated car to my air-conditioned or heated office and the reverse on the trip home. Now, I was outside in all weather, in all seasons of the year, from the sweltering heat of summer to the rare snow of winter. I saw the sunrise in the morning and felt its warmth on my face. I felt blessed.

One spring morning, as I walked the length of my alley, I was overwhelmed by the beauty leafing out around me: the sprouting red oaks, the flowering redbud trees, the wild blue phlox, the sea of Lenten roses I had planted in my yard. Suddenly, I was overcome with emotion. In an instant, it dawned on me: I am not alone. It's not so bad to get old with everything else. I'm part of this changing world with its new life every spring, blossoming, withering, and dying. At that moment, I was so moved that I wept.

Encounter with an Ironman

AFTER ABOUT SIX MONTHS of walking for an hour daily, I met a super-athlete physician at a Leadership Birmingham event. The Leadership Birmingham group met once a month with various professionals around town to learn more about the workings of the city. With Birmingham's dark racial history, I was interested to see that it was money, not a sense of justice or fairness, that brought about a change in racial posturing here in Birmingham. The business community pushed for healthcare, schools, and housing improvements because it helped Birmingham's image.

One day, the Leadership Birmingham group went to Cooper Green, the county hospital, to see what healthcare was offered to the poor. The doctor in the emergency room told us about the hospital and then mentioned having just returned from Hawaii, where he competed in the Ironman Classic. He had swum five miles, run a twenty-six-mile marathon, and biked a hundred miles, all in one day. Inspired, I decided on the spot that I was going to become a mini-Iron person.

First, I went to a bike store. I asked the salesman, "What if you are not sure you can even ride a bike across the room, but want to compete? What bike would you recommend to me?"

The salesman laughed, saying, "I think a mountain bike would fit the bill."

So, I bought a mountain bike and started riding it up and down the alley behind my house. Since I was stronger on one side than the other, I soon realized biking was too dangerous for me. I was too apt to fall. I knew that risking another injury would be a horrendous mistake.

Around the same time, I learned of a fifty-mile swim club at the local gym and signed up with a friend. I felt defeated by the bike, but I was determined to swim the fifty miles. After my first day of walking an hour in the morning and swimming in the evening, I was in so much pain that I could not walk the next day. So, I worked out a schedule.

I would start by swimming every other day and add what I could do without having pain. If all went well, I would increase the amount of swimming time by 10% every week. By doing it this way and stretching after every lap in the pool, I was able to add swimming to my daily exercise routine.

Again and again, I have noticed that when I must start over with an activity or add a new routine, starting at a slow pace and gradually increasing works best for me. Otherwise, too much or too little exercise causes painful spasms in my legs.

To swim in the winter, since the pool was outside, I had to wear my one-piece ski suit from the pool to the dressing room, but I did it. Needless to say, my teenage son, who was exercising in the gym, was mortified to be seen with me. I won't say that I never felt sorry for myself. Everything seemed so much harder for me than it did for everyone else around me. Nevertheless, I kept going.

Given how much I was exercising, I began having illusions that I could enter a fun-run race put on by the gym. I thought to myself, if I'm walking an hour a day, I should be able to do a fun run!

Within seconds of starting the race, the whole group left me behind. I had walked a fairly short distance when a policeman controlling traffic told me, "You will have to walk on the sidewalk, so you don't hold up traffic." When I finally reached the finish line, everyone had gone home. Even the clock was gone. Overwhelmed, I wept tears of frustration and sadness.

But I had learned an important lesson: I did not go alone the next time I did a fun run. I got my son to come with me. After he ran in the 10K race, he lamented how far behind the leaders he was. On the other hand, in my race, I was delighted not to be the last person to finish. Even though I was walking as fast as I could, a group of cardiac patients was talking so much that they were even slower than I was. But what I remember most about that race was what it meant to me to have done this with my son!

Between these fun runs, I read a running magazine. In one edition, a top physician-runner talked about the glories of winning marathons. I shook my head. The joy is not in winning! I wanted to shout. It's about being able to run the race. Over the years, as this physician got older and could not win anymore, I saw that he discovered this for himself.

Next, I entered a fundraiser for the MS Society, walking around Birmingham. For most participants, it was a stroll with stops along the way to eat, drink, or sightsee. For me, it was three and a half hours of pushing myself as hard as I could to reach the end. I was delighted to be able to finish, but once again, I made the mistake of doing it alone. By the end, I felt even more isolated and sorry for myself.

At this point, I had not yet recovered from the fear and shame of my early years with multiple sclerosis. Having friends throughout life is important, and I kept myself much too isolated. Too often, I tended not to participate in activities with others, do things in a group, or even just talk on the phone. I could make myself call someone if I thought I was needed, but I was still too ashamed to share by confiding my own needs. In retrospect, I think I was still affected by depression and did not know how to get the help I needed.

Today, so many people are discovering the glories of doing sports with others who share their affliction. The Dragon Boat Races carried out by breast cancer survivors around the world are the perfect example. These women were once ashamed of having breast cancer yet now relish their success in rowing together, even if they don't win the race.

While I understand why I kept to myself, I also acknowledge it was one of the great mistakes of my life. Everyone with multiple sclerosis, cancer, or any other serious illness feels like a pariah, an outcast. Recognizing that you are not the only one and finding a way to be involved with others can add joy to your life and soften the blow of loss.

At this stage, I was still making foolish mistakes. I wanted so much to be like others who were able to exercise in groups that I tried to walk with a group of women in my neighborhood. I did not even get to the end of the block before they were gone. I turned back and continued walking on my own. For me, the physical challenge of sports felt like a blessing, but I missed out on the human blessing of sharing with others.

Even practicing psychiatry was isolating. Many people like me with chronic illnesses like multiple sclerosis can work, but working consumes all available energy. As for practicing psychiatry, not only can you not discuss your work, but you're likely talked out by the end of the day. I had to make regular luncheon and dinner dates with friends just so I would not become completely disconnected. But I also appreciated how lucky I was to have useful work that made a real difference in people's lives.

It took me seven months, but I did swim fifty miles. By the end, I was walking an hour a day and swimming an hour and twelve minutes—which is how long it took me to swim a mile. As long as I exercised every day and stretched as I went, I no longer had any pain or spasms in my legs. However, the pain would come back if I stopped walking for just two or three days. It took me another year or two of walking and swimming every day before the pain was really gone.

No one had ever told me that I could get rid of the pain completely if I exercised and stretched enough. No one had ever told me I would feel great if I exercised that hard. No one had ever told me that if I worked that hard at exercise, I could manage my weight, end my depression, and even balance my sensitive nervous system.

This discovery changed how I dealt with patients. Never again would I prescribe pills without exploring their level of activity. Realizing the benefits exercise had in controlling my pain and depression, set me up to address chronic pain when I encountered it in my depressed patients.

"*Walking is a man's best medicine.*"
— HIPPOCRATES

"*Strength doesn't come from what you can do. It comes from overcoming the things you once thought you couldn't.*"
— ANONYMOUS

CHAPTER NINE

What Overdoing It Taught Me About Managing Limitations

As I got stronger, I returned to activities I had enjoyed in my youth: hikes with the Sierra Club and outings with the Audubon Society. On one trip to the Bankhead Forest, I was so anxious about being able to keep up that I pushed myself to stay ahead of the group instead of doing what felt good and then sitting down to rest.

The next day, I was in so much pain I knew I was in trouble. I could tell resting for a few days was not going to fix this, so I made an appointment with a doctor at the university's Sports Medicine Clinic. After all, now I was an athlete!

This doctor took one look at me and said, "You need to be at the rehabilitation hospital down the street, not here."

"You don't understand," I said. "I'm an athlete now. I've been walking an hour and swimming a mile every day for over a year. I can't stop now, or I'll get worse."

"Well," he said, "you certainly sound like an athlete!" He looked at my chart. "I will give you a shot of cortisone and turn you over to my physical therapist."

His physical therapist really listened to me. He heard my story of starting to walk and swim, stretching, and pacing myself. I explained, "I walk for an hour, and after about forty minutes, I feel like I could keep going forever."

No medical person had ever listened to me as intently as he did. He smiled. "I have worked with a lot of people with multiple sclerosis. I have never heard any of them say what you just said."

I laughed. "That's probably because none of them have worked as hard as I have." He nodded in assent. I continued, "So, how am I going to manage my exercise when I'm in so much pain?"

"You are not going to stop exercising," he said, "but you are going to change your routine until the pain goes away."

He suggested doing my walking in the pool in addition to swimming laps. In short order, I was better and back to my usual regimen. Still, I had to remember to pace myself and not overdo it. I needed to be my own coach and listen to my own body. It's a lesson that has served me well over the years. Remember, be your own coach! Listen to your body!

Alas, one still has to contend with one's own personality. In my case, this meant my tendency to push too hard and my difficulty asking for help. Years later, my daughter told me, "But Mama, asking for help is one way you make friends!"

Walking in the Alps

THE NEXT SUMMER, I attended the Jung Institute in Zurich, Switzerland, for a two-week conference. A number of the women participants were involved in doing bodywork with patients. Some were physical therapists, and some were trained in Feldenkrais[14] work. The conference was an interesting experience in many ways.

14   Wikipedia.com. The Feldenkrais Method is a type of exercise therapy devised by Israeli Moshé Feldenkrais in the mid-20th century. It is claimed to reorganize

Over the years, I had frequently faced discrimination as a woman in medicine, but this was the first time in a long time I had seen sexism be so blatant. The man running the meeting interacted with the men in the group but completely ignored all the women.

I knew Jung had derived some of his theories from Greek mythology, including his idea about the collective unconscious shared by all humans. After a few days of this meeting, I decided this Jungian[15] approach was less about Greek mythology and more about male-dominated German authoritarianism. Still, the conference provided me with a bonding experience with other women professionals.

One day, several women at the conference planned to walk in the mountains. I thought I could handle it since I had been walking an hour a day, plus swimming. The excursion sounded like fun, so I went along. We were going to walk to a lake, have lunch, perhaps swim, and then return to the other side of the lake. Fortunately, I bought some walking poles before we set off, just in case I needed the extra support.

We were walking uphill in the Alps, and within twenty minutes, I realized I was in trouble. It was a hot day, and I did not have any water. Fortunately, some of the other walkers stayed behind with me and gave me some of theirs. But there was no place to sit down or stretch, so I just had to keep going.

By the time I got to the top of the hill, the others had finished lunch and were preparing to go around the lake and take another

connections between the brain and body, improving body movement and psychological state.

15   Jungian psychology used personality concepts like anima and animus to describe male and female parts of our personality. Plus, archetypes and the collective unconscious, complexes, extraversion and introversion, individuation, the Self, the shadow and synchronicity.

way down. I tried to see if there was a gondola lift I could take down, but it was miles away.

Feeling desperate, I looked for a car or even an ambulance to take me down, but there was nothing in the area. There was no way for me to get back to the car other than returning via the way we had come up. So, by myself, I headed back down.

Going up was easy compared to walking down. I felt like I was going to fall the whole way down. But with the hiking sticks, I made the trip and reached the car before the others were ready to leave. The others were amazed I had made it back in time, but I knew I had been foolish. I had gone without water, without bringing a little seat so I could rest, and without gathering information about the steepness of the climb or ways to get down if it was too much for me. The next day, I was relieved that my right shoulder, from gripping the pole so tight, was the only part of me that hurt.

Still, right there I was faced with failing to deal with loss which we all have to do in the course of a long life. Trying to go along without special preparation was unrealistic and put me at serious risk.

On the bright side, the poles were a real asset. To this day, I walk with two poles so I won't trip. I also added a small metal seat that hangs from around my neck. It has a pocket so I can take water, a book, paints, and some cash. I'm ready to go!

Knowing I had MS, some of the bodywork experts recommended I look into the Feldenkrais method to restore balance to my body when I got home.

Jungian Conference at Home

NOT LONG AFTER I got home, I went to a Jungian conference in Missouri with a group from Birmingham. These were not professionals but people who believed in Jungian ideas. With my medical education and experience, I approached everything discussed at the conference from a different perspective. This experience helped me see how the ideas of groups of people with similar interests may coalesce like devotees of a religion. I had certainly seen this kind of reaction in medicine, where all the doctors tend to buy into the party line and might, therefore, be blind to the limitations of their particular approach.

Sitting in a circle at the first session in Missouri, we were asked to introduce ourselves to the group using one descriptive word. I thought about different possibilities. Being courageous made me feel sad and sorry for myself, but being an athlete made me feel positive and happy. So, despite my limp, I used the word athlete to tell others about myself. I was sure I did not look like an athlete to anyone but me, but defining myself this way felt good.

This experience underscored for me once more the importance of mental attitude in promoting health. Positive attitudes facilitate healing and a return to normal activities, which is needed to get well, whereas negative attitudes can debilitate us. Exercise has given me my life and self-esteem back, in addition to helping me deal with my chronic pain and depression.

In treating patients, I saw how important it was to give them activities beyond taking medications so they could regain control over their lives and facilitate their healing process. Many activities can facilitate having a positive attitude.

I Trip and Fall

AND THEN, ONE DAY, after I walked an hour and swam a mile, I went to the market, tripped over the sidewalk, and broke a bone in my left foot. I was able to walk home but felt very tired. After a nap,

I awoke to find my left foot was massively swollen and painful. I knew I was in trouble.

In the Emergency Department, they x-rayed my foot and put it in a cast. My plan was to ask my secretary to pick me up the next day and take me to the hospital to see patients, but the next morning, I was in too much pain to work.

My mother's nurse/housekeeper brought me food once a day, and within two weeks, my children were home from college. So, I survived. But I was weak as a rag when they took off the cast after six weeks. All my past exercise was for naught. Too late, I realized the stupidity of not having some kind of vigorous exercise to fill in the times of injury or illness. Never again would I let myself go so long without some kind of exercise.

I had to start from the beginning and build up gradually again. But I was lucky. I had already learned the importance of exercise in my life, so I never questioned whether I would get going again. When I did start exercising again, I paced myself, but I never got back to the level I'd been at before breaking my foot. Beware of injury and inactivity. They can really set you back.

After that, I bought a machine to exercise my back, abdominals, arms, and legs in a sitting position. I also asked one of the trainers at my gym to design an exercise program I could do at home, sitting in a chair and lying in bed. He gave me exercises to do in bed (leg lifts, clam shells, etc.), sitting in a chair watching TV (arm exercises and knee lifts), standing at the counter waiting for the teakettle to boil (squats, push-ups, and dancing in place), etc.

This routine gave me a weight-training program using my own arms and legs as weights and encouraged me to move vigorously in bed or a chair to get an aerobic workout. It also taught me the importance of building exercise into my daily activities in addition to a daily exercise routine.

Movement is exercise, so put on your favorite music and move while lying flat or sitting in a chair. To this day, I have exercises I do while waiting for a kettle to boil, watching television, or riding in an elevator. Squats are a special magic.

MS Progress

As I MOVED INTO my early forties, I had more episodes of multiple sclerosis. New symptoms might appear along with the numbness and tingling I'd had in the past, or old symptoms might reappear by themselves. One time, I lost hearing in my left ear. There were periods of increased unsteadiness and periods of having funny pains, called dysesthesia, like a burning sensation in my scalp, which felt numb to the touch. With each episode, I felt scared and sorry for myself, especially because I was alone. But even though my trouble walking never went away, most symptoms did improve over time.

One time, I got dizzy and lost my sense of taste. Food was taste-less. I could not even appreciate its texture. I thought how foolish I'd been all my life, berating myself for eating too much food when I should have been celebrating my great sense of taste!

Later, I learned a friend had also become dizzy and lost her sense of taste after having the flu. She went to her internist and got medicine for vertigo, while I did not. After this episode, I realized multiple sclerosis might not be the cause of everything. And resolved to see a doctor if new symptoms appeared, just to be sure it was not something else.

Fortunately, my taste came back. I was once again able to cele-brate my enjoyment of food. I decided weight was just something I had to contend with and stopped berating myself for eating too much.

*"The deeper that sorrow carves into your being,
the more joy you can contain."*
— KHALIL GIBRAN

*"Live to inspire, and one day people will say,
because of you, I didn't give up"* –
— UNKNOWN

*"The best way to find yourself is to lose
yourself in the service of others."*
— MAHATMA GANDHI

CHAPTER TEN

Giving Back—Learning How Helping Others is a Constructive Way to Help Yourself

In 1988, I was now in private practice but still teaching medical students about addiction in their sophomore pharmacology course, and also about physician impairment[16] in their junior Introduction to Medicine course. I agreed to serve as Psychiatrist on the Advisory Board of the Multiple Sclerosis Society.

I walked into the first meeting wondering if everyone in the room knew that I had MS. Could everyone tell just by seeing me walk with a limp? There were patient advisors on the board who talked openly about having the disease, but I didn't say a word about my own situation. Truthfully, I was afraid I might burst into tears. Maybe everyone assumed that having multiple sclerosis was why I had been invited to join the Advisory Board in the first place, even though most of the other doctors on the Advisory Board did not have MS. At that point, I still viewed MS as a stigma that would set

---

16 Physician impairment was a euphemism for drug and alcohol problems even though physicians might become impaired for other reasons.

me up to be pitied or easily dismissed by others. My fear made me my own worst enemy.

However, it was at this meeting that I met the Neurology Department's new Chairman and multiple sclerosis specialist, Dr. Eric Martin. He talked about the clinic he was running to assist neurologists all over the state with making diagnoses and managing patients with severe cases of multiple sclerosis.

At this time, in the 1980s, because there were no MRIs to aid with diagnosis, patients with symptoms of MS but no physical signs were often thought to be malingering.[17] As a result, many neurologists around the state sent anyone they suspected of having MS to Dr. Martin's clinic. Dr. Martin also saw patients with severe cases of multiple sclerosis and made treatment suggestions for them. His work intrigued me, and I volunteered to work in his clinic one half-day a week.

However, as my first day at the clinic approached, I began having second thoughts. I could not help but think, what if I see how I might end up and can't deal with it? Multiple sclerosis is a terrifying disease, capable of robbing one of all neurologic functions. I was scared every time I got a new symptom, but so far, I had been able to tell myself I was likely to get better. In this clinic, however, I would see the full range of this dreaded illness. I considered changing my mind, but Dr. Martin was eager for me to come.

I began my tenure in the clinic by following Dr. Martin on his rounds with patients. After he had completed his physical exam, I would stay and talk with the patient. This became my favorite way of interviewing patients because I could watch their interaction with

---

17 Pretending to be ill to escape duty or work.

Dr. Martin and the other physicians and see what I might add to the initial evaluation.

Joining the clinic staff was an important step for me. Almost immediately, I felt a sense of relief. Having had MS for twenty years, it looked to me as if I had already survived this disease. I felt deep compassion for the patients in this clinic, who ran the gamut from having a few sensory symptoms to those who were totally paralyzed.

But none of these patients had had MS for as long as fifteen years, much less twenty years, as I had. True, I had some permanent damage from multiple sclerosis that affected my gait. But I was walking for an hour a day in the morning and swimming for over an hour in the evening, and I had not had a new MS episode for several years. I felt I had already survived the worst of the disease.

In addition, watching Dr. Martin interview and examine patients helped me to see why neurologists often failed to help their patients. If a neurologist couldn't find any signs of damage to the brain or spinal cord on the physical exam, he tended to dismiss the patient's symptoms as being due to anxiety, depression, or faking.

Having MS myself, I knew that someone with sensory symptoms from multiple sclerosis might not have any physical signs but could still be very anxious about what was happening to them. This had been the case with me for the first ten years. During that time, I was both anxious and depressed. So, I knew that patients were more likely to be anxious because of the MS symptoms. In fact, they were more likely to be anxious and depressed than someone without those sensory changes.

This was an epiphany to me. Because of my experience with MS, I was able to observe a major flaw in how physicians viewed physical illness when symptoms of anxiety or depression were present in a patient. The same could be true of behavior changes in patients who were confused by delirium but too often dismissed.

A Series of Epiphanies

I LEARNED ABOUT ANXIETY during my training in psychiatry. However, my training took place at a time when psychiatrists did not fully understand all the manifestations of anxiety and still believed that only women and the feeble-minded showed signs of hysteria or pseudo-neurologic symptoms.[18]

I was taught that hysterical symptoms were consistently associated with secondary gain—that is, doctors believed hysterical symptoms were an act that patients put on to get attention and to manipulate their families and their doctors. As a result, most physicians despised "hysterics" and passed them off to psychiatry as soon as they could. That meant these doctors failed to explore the patient's complaint with the same care they might explore a more obvious physical symptom.

At that time, doctors did not realize that these pseudo-symptoms were an unconscious way to deal with anxiety, most often seen when there was actual damage to the brain from MS, a tumor, or some other physical problem. Doctors failed to see that these symptoms were telling them as much about what was going on with their patients as any physical sign. Instead, they tended to dismiss such complaints and such patients, making them less able to be helpful to that patient.

Ironically, the first patient I saw with hysteria as a psych resident was a man. He was described as a "classical case of hysteria" by one of my professors. The patient had come into the ER saying he had

18   Hysterical symptoms or pseudo-neurological signs are conditions that look like a neurological problem, but don't follow the usual anatomical rule.

tetanus. Because he was flailing about, the ER sent him to psychiatry, where my professor said it was a "classical" case of hysteria, a form of anxiety, and sent him home with tranquilizers.

Days later, when the man returned to the ER, even the students could see that this man did indeed have tetanus. This patient may, in fact, have been flailing about as a symptom of anxiety when he first arrived, but underlying the flailing about, there was a very real problem that had not yet been discovered.

In truth, I have never seen a patient with anxiety manifested as a pseudo-neurologic symptom who did not have something physically wrong. That case taught me an important lesson. Never again would I dismiss a pseudo-symptom without looking for something physically wrong.

The next patient I saw after that, who was believed to be suffering from hysteria, was admitted to my service one Sunday afternoon to be treated for worsening depression. The patient told me she had hysteria.

As I looked at her lying in bed, she told me, "My husband was talking about divorce when the paralysis first appeared. He would have left me if I'd been able to walk and take care of myself. I have had hysteria for about twenty years."

Among other things, her legs were frozen in a bent position. She had not walked for years. I knew hysteria did not cause this kind of paralysis and contracture. Fresh from my patient with tetanus, I went looking for a physical cause for her paralysis.

A lumbar tap showed this patient had a previously undiagnosed case of multiple sclerosis. A psychiatrist had treated her for hysteria for twenty years, and all that time, she believed her paralysis was caused by fear that her husband would leave her.

The look in her eyes when I told her that she had MS told me a great deal. She wept with relief. "I always felt guilty, thinking I had somehow manipulated my husband into staying in this marriage."

There was still no treatment for MS, so having the correct diagnosis did not help this patient function better, but at least she and her husband were able to start the rest of their lives from a different perspective.

Around the same time, another patient with multiple sclerosis and 'hysteria' came to see me. Immediately, I recognized her. I had once treated this woman for alcoholism. Before seeing me this time, she had spent six weeks in the hospital with what her chart described as "pseudo-paralysis," an anxiety-driven paralysis.

"My doctors said they could not tell me when the paralysis might come back!" She paused in her tale and added in almost a whisper, "I'm scared to death my multiple sclerosis is getting worse."

I directed her to a chair. "How long has it been since you had a new MS symptom?" I asked her.

She thought for a moment, then said, "It's been over twenty years."

"That's good," I said. "It means your multiple sclerosis is not progressing. Now tell me, when do you have these symptoms like those you were having in the hospital?"

I could see her concentrating as she thought. "I get these symptoms when I fight with my husband and especially when I don't get enough support from him." She paused. "When I feel overwhelmed." She looked at me directly. "And I guess when I start drinking too much," she added sheepishly.

"Wonderful!" I told her. "Now you know what you can do to address these particular episodes. Getting back into AA will help you with the drinking. Get your husband to go back to counseling with that minister who was helping you. Finally, ask your family and friends to give you additional support so you have the help you need, so you don't get overwhelmed. Be sure to ask them for specific things like going to the market or preparing a meal, so they know what to expect, and you don't set yourself up for disappointment."

We talked some more, and she went away smiling. She now knew her multiple sclerosis was not getting worse, and she had a plan to address the symptoms she feared. This patient's physical problem, multiple sclerosis, was already known, so my job was limited to unraveling the situations that triggered her anxiety symptoms. This is not something any test can reveal.

This was further confirmation of my observation that patients with anxiety and sensory symptoms are likely to have something physically wrong that just has not reached their level of consciousness yet or shown up on a test or physical exam. However, their unconscious mind is aware of a problem and is reacting to it.

Frequently, I observed that patients might have hysteria or pseudo-neurologic symptoms to protect themselves from injury or from being overwhelmed. But once the physical cause is found, the pseudo-symptoms always make sense in a patient's life.

The neurology doctors in the multiple sclerosis clinic were not focusing on the right things. I knew that anxiety meant someone was more likely to have MS or something physically wrong, not less. Someone with sensory symptoms and anxiety merited a more aggressive approach to evaluation, not one that was less robust.

Since I was more determined to look for physical problems than were the neurologists, I was able to demonstrate physical problems on EEG or CT scans that the others missed when they assumed the symptoms were "merely due to anxiety or depression." I recalled my early "escalator phobia" before I realized I simply could not locate my foot in space. I could tell something was wrong—just not what.

Another Epiphany

OVER AND OVER, I observed the physicians at the clinic having trouble understanding the connection between depression or manifestation of anxiety, conversion disorders, psychological manifestations, and physical symptoms or illness. Neurologists tended to think they were either one or the other rather than recognizing that both were likely to be present.

Perhaps that was why I always knew what was wrong with a patient sent to me for evaluation who had already consulted several other doctors, especially neurologists and psychiatrists. All of these patients had something physically wrong, either known or unknown, and all had some manifestation of anxiety or depression, which was confusing the picture. The physical problem may have been known since childhood, like polio, but only became a problem later when the support system failed. Or the physical problem may be a brain tumor that has not yet been uncovered, but the unconscious knows it is there.

The most dramatic example of physicians dismissing possible physical causes underlying a behavior change was a patient sent to my office by one of the neurologists for treatment of depression.

"The physical examination was normal, so I think he must be depressed," the neurologist told me.

This patient had once been a pilot and had formerly been a very responsible man. Yet over the course of a year, he had withdrawn from his work, done less and less at home, and was currently spending all his time in bed. In the previous six months, his wife had started divorce proceedings against him.

The divorce was nearly finalized when the wife made an appointment for her husband to see me. In fact, he missed his first appointment, and I had to get the full story from his wife.

I arranged for this former pilot to be admitted to the hospital and ordered an EEG and a CT scan, which was all that was available to me at the time. After the tests, the neurologist called me and said, "The EEG looks like a metabolic storm." Metabolic storm is a term for a chemical storm in the brain.

"I thought he had a brain tumor," I replied. "He's been getting progressively worse over the past year."

The neurologist called me back the next morning. "He has a brain tumor, all right. It's huge. It looks like a meningioma, a non-malignant tumor."

"So, he'll be all right once they take it out?" I asked.

"I don't know. This tumor is so large, he'll probably have some permanent damage."

After the man's divorce was final, he moved to Charleston to live with his father and have the surgery.

This man's plight so grieved me that I found myself writing poetry! It was such a tragedy.

I decided then to do more teaching with young doctors—both medical interns and residents and neurological residents—to be sure that all learned the importance of treating symptoms of anxiety, depression, and behavior change with the same respect as belly pain or paralysis. They are all clues to what is going on with the patient: a clue to finding the physical cause. Doing this work, I just felt blessed to be stable enough to be helpful to others.

Dr. Martin was chairman of the Department of Neurology at the University. While I was working in his MS Clinic, he was asked to take over the Department of Psychiatry as well as Neuro. He told me he would only accept the offer to head both departments if I would manage the Department of Psychiatry for him. I was stunned. Since the previous Chairman of Psychiatry had fired me, this seemed like the ultimate affirmation.

I hadn't seen a neurologist in years. I did not see what they had to offer me. However, Interferon appeared on the market in 1994 as the first real treatment for multiple sclerosis. Dr. Martin was one of the doctors evaluating the drug for the entire nation. I decided to ask him if he would see me and determine if I should take this new medicine. Still, it took all the bravery I could muster just to call him up and ask him to take me on as a patient.

"Sure, I'd be glad to see you," he said. "Just send me your latest MRI."

"I've never had an MRI," I countered.

"Never had an MRI? I will make the arrangements and get you in after that." He ordered two MRIs, one of my head and one of my neck. Plus, he added evoked potentials. These are special tests to evaluate damage to my eyes and ears.

As reassuring and bolstering as all my interactions with Dr. Martin had been in the MS Clinic, I felt terrified as my actual appointment with him approached. I'd been able to hide my insecurity and deep feelings of vulnerability in his clinic because I was focused on the patients and felt my contributions were useful to them. Focusing on others always helped me deal with anxiety about myself. I did not realize it then, but helping others can be an unconscious defense mechanism to help deal with anxiety, as well as a great coping mechanism we can plan into our lives.

As I thought about taking Interferon, I remembered what my

own patients had said about taking it: they were sick for days every week. Did I really want to put myself in that situation? I did not want to feel bad all the time, as I had shifted my focus to what was going well in my life.

I thought about my daily exercise routine: first, walking for an hour in the morning. How great it felt to be up with the sun every day, walking along swinging my arms, listening to great music, stopping for a sip of hot tea as I walked another length of my alley.

I thought about my sense of triumph as I swam in the pool every night. I had added moves like slaloming in the pool. It felt like being on the ski slopes. There was a lot I could not do, but I had mastered my routine, and I felt good in my body and spirit most of the time. After walking forty minutes in the morning, I felt so good I could have gone on forever! Did I really want to subject myself to being part of a medical study and feel bad about not being able to exercise as much?

I will never forget the shock I had when Dr. Martin pulled out my chart to look at the test results and said: "The tests show you have chronic-progressive multiple sclerosis. Your tests show you have had optic neuritis in both eyes, so in addition to problems with your gait, your hearing has been affected, too."

As Dr. Martin started to speak again, I forced myself to listen.

"Unfortunately, at this time, we're only studying the effects of Interferon[19] on patients with relapsing-remitting multiple sclerosis," he said as he took a breath. "If anything else comes along, I will let you know."

I was stunned. I felt like I'd been hammered. Why is he telling me I have the worst kind of multiple sclerosis if he has nothing to

---

19   This was 1996 and Interferon had just been identified as useful in treating MS.

offer me? I'd known for twenty-five years that I had MS. Alas, this was not the first nor last time I was about to decide doctors could be as destructive as they might be helpful.

"If you stumble, make it part of the dance."
— UNKNOWN

"As in the inflammations and fevers of physical illness,
what looks like trouble may be the very process by
which healing takes place. As we become better
able to endure life's slings and arrows, our
coping mechanisms mature, and vice versa."
— GEORGE E. VAILLANT, TRIUMPHS OF EXPERIENCE:
THE MEN OF THE HARVARD GRANT STUDY

CHAPTER ELEVEN

Revisiting My Diagnosis and the Role of the Doctor

In 2004, I started having pain in my right knee. I went to the doctor, who informed me, "You have a torn medial meniscus. We need to do surgery to take out loose pieces."

Shortly after the procedure, I could tell I'd made a mistake: all I wanted to do was lie in bed and not move. In time, I realized the surgery had precipitated an episode of depression and sought help. In addition, my knee was much more unstable than it had been before surgery.

Eventually, I needed knee replacement surgery because I was falling and afraid I might injure myself. When my other knee started hurting, I went back to the doctor. Again, I had a torn meniscus, but this time, I refused surgery and decided to use exercise to deal with the problem. I know that joint is more vulnerable because it slips at times, but doing daily squats, leg lifts, and walking has helped me stay strong and pain-free in that leg.

Before the knee replacement, I looked for a doctor to help me stay physically strong in the course of having MS. I went to see a physical medicine specialist, thinking that physical therapy would be his focus. Rather than address my stretching and exercise routine, this doctor ordered two MRIs of my neck and brain, plus conduction studies of my wrist for carpal tunnel syndrome and elbow for my ulnar tunnel syndrome, and then sent me to a neurologist who specialized in multiple sclerosis. All these diagnoses I already knew I had, and I received no new help with my struggles.

It had been more than twenty years since I'd seen a neurologist and more than twenty years since I'd had a new symptom of MS, so I was not sure what this neurologist had to offer me, but I decided to go to find out if it would be safe for me to get flu shots. Thirty years before, a flu shot had precipitated a vision loss in my left eye, so I had stayed away from flu shots after that.

This new neurologist, Dr. Barth, had served with me on the MS Society Medical Advisory Board years earlier. I also recognized one of the nurses who had served with me in the MS clinic when I worked with Dr. Martin.

Dr. Barth greeted me warmly, took my history, and examined my records. "It says here you have chronic-progressive multiple sclerosis, but you have done so well," he said. "I think you must actually have relapsing-remitting multiple sclerosis. It just did not remit." That is to say, go away.

Good news! I thought. He thinks I'm doing well!

Having seen my latest MRIs, he said, "You seem to be stable, so I don't think you need any medication for MS." He then began telling me about his research into a new medication for MS.

Finally—someone who doesn't just want to put me on pills.

"What symptom bothers you the most?" he asked.

"Fatigue," I said without hesitation.

"We've been using Provigil, a stimulant, for that," he said. "We've had good results. Would you like to try some?"

I nodded. Finally, I would have a medicine to help with fatigue and also treat depression when the grey fog overtook me.

Initially, I found taking a stimulant every day caused me too many problems. I felt wired all the time and had to sleep it off when I stopped. Instead, taking a smaller dose of Provigil if I needed energy to be with my grandchildren or go out in the evening worked well. Most of the time, however, I just used coffee, daily exercise, and naps to deal with fatigue. I also took a small dose of Provigil when I felt stuck in depression. It turns out that stimulants like Provigil are especially effective at treating depression precipitated by surgery or illness like MS.

During the interview, I noticed Dr. Barth used the same disability scale they had used twenty-five years before. He never once asked me anything about exercise. Like the previous MS specialist, he showed no interest in why I might be doing so well. The nurse routinely asked me to rate my pain level.

My Next Encounter

ABOUT TEN YEARS LATER, my internist retired, and I had to find a new doctor. This new internist wanted me to check in with Dr. Barth. By then, I'd had multiple sclerosis for nearly fifty years. Sitting in the general waiting area for this appointment, I thought about how well I'd been doing and what might have saved me.

The nurse who called me in directed me to an exam room and asked me to fill out a sheet of information about myself and my condition. I was not taking Provigil regularly, only when I needed it to function or was too tired. As far as my overall function went, nothing had really changed. My walking was more labored since I had not been walking as much. I'd been sick in the spring and needed antibiotics four times. As a result, I had not been exercising and stretching as much as usual.

Two young men came in to examine me. "I'm Dr. Solars," one said. "I'm Dr. Barth's assistant."

The other man introduced himself as a neurology resident. The assistant examined me.

Then, Dr. Solars said, "Dr. Barth will be in to see you in a minute."

When Dr. Barth appeared, he said, "You're weaker. I want you to get an MRI and either get you on MS medicine or have surgery."

I looked at him with astonishment. He examined me but did not take any history, which would have told him I'd been sick all spring with one infection after another. Sickness of any kind brings out my MS symptoms. Also, I hadn't been exercising and stretching as much as usual. Plus, I had been singing in the choir for Easter. All that standing up and sitting down always made my walking worse. This doctor had never once asked me about exercise or stretching, even though I'd asked him for a referral to physical therapy from time to time when I saw him. His nurse faithfully asked me to rate my pain level from one to ten, but there was never a question about exercise.

"Well, I'm not going to have surgery or take medicine, so there's no point in doing an MRI. If I'm worse the next time I come, I will do it then." I was sure I could exercise and regain my strength.

At that, I thought he would tell me to come back in three months. Instead, he said, "Let me see you in a year."

I wanted to say, "So, you're not very concerned about the change in my status!" But I did not. Did I hold back because of my early training? Did I think saying such a thing wouldn't be ladylike? Was I afraid that challenging him would alienate him? I hadn't even asked him why he wanted the tests.

When I got home, I was furious. I was mad at myself for not asking enough questions and mad at the doctor, too. The stupidity of his not asking why my walking might be worse and not taking a history focused on why I might be worse seemed obvious.

Without exercise, I get weaker and feeble and, of course, gain weight. My activity level does decrease when I'm injured, go through periods of sickness or depression, struggle with bad weather, or even get overwhelmed with the holidays. But I always get back to exercising again because I know it's my lifeline.

As I waited to see Dr. Barth, I thought back on my various encounters with doctors over the years. I thought about what Dr. Barth had said when I first saw him. He saw my chart and said I had the worst kind of MS: Chronic Progressive. "But I think you must actually have the best kind of MS: relapsing-remitting. It just did not remit (go away)."

Why had I not asked him at the time, "What if I have chronic-progressive MS and it just did not progress because I have been doing such vigorous exercise, especially in my forties and fifties?" I had never thought about it that way before, but after all this time, it seemed logical.

I couldn't help but wonder if I *did* have relapsing-remitting MS. I certainly would not have thought it was chronic-progressive MS because I was so stable.

Galvanized by my fury, I got on the internet and searched for "effects of exercise on the inflammatory and degenerative phases of multiple sclerosis."

MS has two phases: the inflammatory phase, when lesions form in the brain and spinal cord, and the degenerative phase, when patients become weaker from inactivity.

To my delight, I found that scientists had finally done the research to show what I already suspected: exercise treats both phases of multiple sclerosis. It reverses the inflammatory damage to the nervous system and prevents inactivity from weakening me.

It appears that exercise increases Brain-Derived Neurotrophic Factor (BDNF),[20] which is neuroprotective. So, exercise is crucial for preventing the progression of disease. Just as depression can shrink the corpus callous in the brain, and that can be reversed by anti-depressants or exercise, so too exercise changes the brain in MS. It was once thought that exercise heated up the body and brought out more MS symptoms, but now we know that inactivity will actually speed up the disease. I copied the articles to take to Dr. Barth the next time I saw him.[21]

You Will Hurt If You Don't Move and Stretch

THAT WAS THE YEAR my husband completed his novel, *Andre's Reboot.* Facing my next appointment with Dr. Barth, I found myself working on a memoir of my life with MS—but only after exercising first thing in the morning.

My husband, however, sat at his desk day after day, bent over his computer. By the time spring arrived, his back hurt. He went to

20   Matthew T. Schmolesky, David L. Webb,1, and Rodney A. Hansen, "The Effects of Aerobic Exercise Intensity and Duration on Levels of Brain-Derived Neurotrophic Factor in Healthy Men," J Sports Sci Med, 2013, (3): 502–511.

21   Briggs, Nicole, "Effects of Exercise on the Progression of Multiple Sclerosis," Physician's Assistant Program Capstones, 2020: 47, scholarlycommons.pacific. edu/pa-capstones/47.

see his back doctor, who had given him spinal blocks[22] with general anesthesia in the past and told him he could have up to three a year if needed. He recommended having a spinal block.

I was shocked. "I refuse to take you in for another spinal block," I blurted out. "You have a chronic back condition. You need to manage that problem with exercise and stretching daily. Instead, you have hunched over your computer all day for months, with no exercise or stretching. No wonder you hurt!"

Fortunately, I was vindicated when he forced himself to mow the lawn again, and the pain disappeared. I'm almost sure his doctor did not ask him what he had been doing and how often he exercised and stretched.

The Cost of Waiting to Hear About Test Results

THE NEGATIVE EFFECT OF waiting to hear the worst from test results is not negligible. When Dr. Barth wanted me to have an MRI to assess my increased weakness, I declined because I thought I knew why I was weaker. But as time passed and the date of my next appointment eventually got pushed back to a year and a half later, I began to worry.

Instead of thinking I was successfully managing my weakness and periodic pain with exercise and stretching, I became discouraged and fearful I might have secondary progressive MS. I began worrying that I was in denial about the state of my MS. How could I not be scared when I realized I was part of a medical system that was too often not connected to my needs, my symptoms, or my concerns.

If I fit into their system of evaluation and treatment, I might or might not get any help, but I certainly wasn't going to get the encouragement I needed to continue doing what I'd had to do to survive.

In my youth, I'd had confidence in my ability to work things out, but as I got older, I did not always feel so secure.

This whole situation with Dr. Barth reminded me of the time in my fifties when I developed pain in my left eye. My medical doctor wanted me to see a specialist, a neuro-ophthalmologist. I had to wait three months for the appointment. When I arrived, the staff ran me through a full range of eye tests, all of which came back normal.

When the doctor finally appeared, he said in a tone both impatient and surly, "What are you doing here? All your tests are normal!"

As he turned abruptly to leave, I said, "I have had optic neuritis in my left eye in the past, and now that eye hurts."

He stopped and turned back to examine my left eye again to make sure they had not missed something. "Nothing wrong," he said, turning to leave again.

"So, why do I hurt?" I asked.

"I don't know," he said on his way out the door.

"So, when should I come back?" I called after him.

"Five years."

It had been five years since my last normal exam.

No one in the eye doctor's office ever took a medical history or even asked me why I had come in. No one said, "Tell me when this pain began. What is it like? Does it come and go, or is it present all the time? What makes it worse? Better? What have you tried to make it better? What other health problems do you have? Any migraines or headaches? MS? What medications do you take? Does this medicine cause eye pain?"

I had to figure out on my own that the pain was caused by the medication I was taking for depression, Prozac.

Dr. Barth routinely asked questions from a standard disability scale to see if my body was getting weaker. It never changed. On every visit, he wanted me to rate my pain level from one to ten. But nowhere, ever, was there a question about exercise. While depression is very common in patients with MS, even caused by MS, there was no attempt to be sure I was aware of depression and getting the proper treatment when it occurred.

All too often, our modern medical system often fails to address why the patient comes to the doctor in the first place. Remember, it is anxiety or fear about what is happening to us that takes us to the doctor, not bleeding, pain, or vomiting. Fear about what a symptom means drives us to make an appointment or dash to the ER. Doctors are trained to rule out life-threatening situations, but running tests to do so may not address a particular patient's concerns or needs at a particular time.

Although the evidence-based medicine (EBM) method was an attempt to bypass the prejudices and ignorance of individual medical doctors by basing therapy only on scientific evidence—that is, tests—the designers of this method overlooked the basic needs of patients coming into the office in the first place: to allay their concerns and fears.

In addition to the biases inherent in every test-based encounter, as well as every scientific experiment, failure to address the patient's concerns means medicine is an expensive exercise in futility for many people seeking care.

Medicine is too often focused on its own agenda, rather than all the factors that may play on a patient's difficulty. Increased weakness in someone with MS may mean the MS is active needing modern medicine or may mean bones are impinging on the spinal cord, but it might mean MS depression has caused the patient to be weaker because of decreased activity, infections, or other illnesses have led to decreased activity.

Always testing rather than taking a history also overlooks the benefit of making a diagnosis based on information from the patient rather than numbers from one or more tests. My doctors' insistence on running tests rather than talking with me not only brought me a lot of grief and anxiety about what might be happening to me, but it also cost a lot of money to run tests that ultimately failed to address my problem in any way.

I did agree to the MRI when I next saw Dr. Barth. I had to wait weeks to get the results, which showed no MS activity or pressure on my spinal cord, so there was no need for medicine or surgery. So, *no one did anything useful about my problem.*

I gave Dr. Barth the articles I had copied bout the effect of exercise on both the inflammatory and degenerative phases of MS, but he dismissed the subject by saying he already knew about these findings. And that was the end of the matter.

Discovering the Natural Way to Retard Illness

No one ever told me about the importance and power of exercise in treating the inflammatory and degenerative effects of multiple sclerosis. When I was first diagnosed, doctors did not know about this kind of treatment for arresting the disease's progress.

When I finally saw Dr. Martin about taking Interferon, I had been exercising two hours a day for several years and had not had a new MS episode in that time. The old damage did not go away, and it got worse anytime I had an infection or other physical stress, but after that, I did not develop any new symptoms of multiple sclerosis.

When doctors finally offered me medication for multiple sclerosis about thirty years into my illness, I turned it down. I knew I did not do well with the side effects of medicine.

I have a clumsy walk, which puts strain on my body. I've had to have a knee replacement because I was falling backward and afraid I might hurt myself. I have a severely collapsed arch on my left foot, which the orthopedist said would eventually need surgery, but I've found I can manage with exercise and stretching.

I have learned the benefit of movement, exercise, along with stretching to manage pain in lieu of surgery.[23] When regular stretching is not sufficient, a tennis ball run under my foot or placed under a tight calf muscle can stretch the muscle and free me from pain again. These days, there are even special vibrators for tight muscles.

Today, we know exercise treats both the inflammatory and degenerative aspects of multiple sclerosis and other neurological conditions like Parkinson's disease. I was just lucky to have stumbled onto exercise and stretching as a way to get my life back so young.

When I saw the effect vigorous exercise had on my chronic pain and depression, it changed the way I practiced medicine. Never again would I give patients medication for depression or anxiety without encouraging them to exercise as well. It also led me to work more with medical patients suffering from depression and, ultimately, chronic pain.

I tell this story in my first two books, *Heal: A Psychiatrist's Inspiring Story of What It Takes to Recover from Chronic Pain, Depression, and Addiction.* And, *What Stands in the Way and Heal Thyself: What You Can Do to Recover from Chronic Pain, Depression, and Addiction.* In these books, I describe in detail the myriad ways

23   In 2010, during a visit to Northern Ireland for the summer, I started to have pain in my left foot, the one that collapses due to weakness from MS. I didn't know what to do. We were used to walking for hours around the town of Port Rush, stopping along the way to have rhubarb pie with whipped cream and a pot of strong English tea. I could hardly walk across the room. Fortunately, I could Google "foot pain" and get some suggestions. The combination of going up on my toes ten times every time I washed my hands, plus stretching my heel off a step several times an hour, let me stretch out the pain and keep going.

natural therapies like exercise can benefit those with chronic pain and depression.

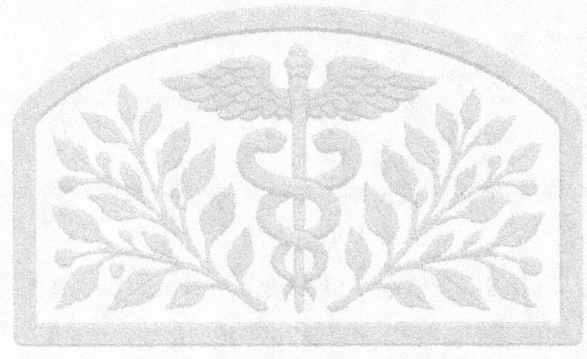

PART TWO

MEDICINE'S WAR ON NATURAL THERAPIES

HOW I DISCOVERED THE IMPORTANCE OF
NATURAL THERAPIES

In Part Two, I will explore discoveries I made about alternative forms of therapy in the course of living my life and working with patients. I start with what I learned about the failure to recognize the connection between depression and chronic pain, or the presence of depression in those patients who are non-compliant with treatment. Then I describe what I discovered about natural therapies in the course of treating chronic pain, the history of medicine's war on natural therapies, what's involved in healing and the placebo effect, AND how food fits into natural therapies.

"A physician is obligated to consider more than a diseased organ, more than even the whole man—he must view the man in his world."
— HARVEY CUSHING

"It is found easier, by the short-sighted victims of disease, to palliate their torments by medicine, than to prevent them by regimen."
— PERCY BYSSHE SHELLEY

Chronic Pain Became the Vehicle for Understanding the Importance of Alternative or Natural Therapies: The Role of Depression and Other Emotions in a Medical Setting

By 1990, my children were grown, and I sought ways to expand my professional activities. So, when the medical director of the county hospital offered me an opportunity to teach medical students and young doctors about the psychiatric areas most seen in medical practice, that is, pain, anxiety, depression, suicide, addiction, and organic mental syndromes, I jumped at the chance. I would also see depressed patients in his medical clinic one day a week.

From my earliest days teaching medical students in their sophomore year pharmacology course about the therapeutic uses of drugs of abuse, it was obvious to me that doctors were not getting the right training to help them understand and manage the psychiatric problems that are part of everyday practice in medicine and surgery. That is, the medical students were not being taught about the anxiety, depression, and suicidal thinking that must be part of every serious illness or injury.

They were not hearing enough about the management of acute and chronic pain. They were not hearing how best to use opiates for the management of acute or chronic pain, nor how to handle the threat of addiction when patients are prescribed opiates, tranquilizers, or stimulants. And they needed to understand how confusion or delirium can result from any medical illness or surgical procedure.

In my experience, psychiatric training for medical students was usually focused on treating schizophrenic patients on the inpatient psychiatric ward. When I was at the county hospital, Cooper Green, I would get to focus on bread-and-butter psychiatric issues that physicians should know how to recognize and manage every day.

As we sat in front of a fire in my living room, I remember the medical director's words now seared into my memory: "Your profession is bankrupt," he said—meaning psychiatry. "Patients who need you are either seeing other doctors like me or are wandering the streets without access to care."

I had been working with him on the homeless population, many of whom suffered from schizophrenia. He wanted me to teach on morning rounds with the medical staff once a week, followed by a two-hour teaching session with the medical students. Then, in the afternoon, I would see depressed patients in the medical clinic.

Little did I anticipate how many more problems I would unearth: depression and suicide attempts being missed, and chronic pain getting too many opiates. The connection between pain and depression was a new one to me, but it hit me in the face from day one.

The Connection Between Pain and Depression

MY VERY FIRST PATIENT in the medical clinic was a woman who had multiple health issues. Now, she was responsible for caring for all her older relatives. She was clearly depressed, but looking at her chart, I noticed she was also suffering from back pain. Fresh from my own experience with pain, I zeroed in on that complaint.

"What is the doctor doing for your pain?" I asked.

"He gives me opiates," she said, "but I can't afford them most of the time."

"Have you been to physical therapy?" I asked, suspicious of the opiate prescription.

"The doctor did send me," she said, "but it made my pain worse and was expensive, so I did not go back."

I found myself feeling angry that this woman had been denied the simple suggestions that could change her life. Although I was seeing her for depression and planned to give her the antidepressant medication I'd brought with me to treat depression, I couldn't hear this woman's statement and not tell her about my own experience with pain and what had saved me.

So, in the course of five minutes, I told her my story. Then, firmly wedded to the idea that antidepressants were needed to treat her depression, I made an appointment for her to return in two weeks so I could check on her medicine.

As was true with so many patients at Cooper Green, I did not see her again for a year. When she returned, I did not recognize her. At our first meeting, she had looked like she held the weight of the world on her shoulders, which indeed she did. Now, she sat up straight and looked confident.

"I know you don't remember me," she said. "I couldn't come back to see you last year because I had too many problems, but I did what you said. And it changed my life." She continued, "In the beginning, I was so wobbly, I had to have someone walk on each side of me. But I did walk every day, and now, I'm walking two miles a day with a friend. It's the best part of my life."

Too often, doctors think it's easier to prescribe pills than to spend enough time to get the patient moving in a different direction. Did my obvious distress over her plight make the difference? Did sharing my own experience give her the impetus to really do what I suggested, whereas telling her she needed exercise would not? Was she just desperate enough to try anything? I don't know, but exercise transformed her life, resolved her depression as well as her pain, and gave her some control over her difficult life.

Treating medical clinic patients with depression helped me see the connection between chronic pain as a symptom of depression, which I had not appreciated before I went to Cooper Green. Even though I had suffered from depression and exercise had resolved my depression as well as my pain, I had not made that connection myself. It seemed nearly everyone in the medical clinic sent to me for depression had some kind of chronic pain as a symptom of the depression!

Estimates run as high as 75% of those with chronic pain are depressed. Even soldiers returning from Iraq with PTSD/depression, though they'd never had a physical injury, had chronic pain!

Thanks to my own experience with chronic pain and how limited the standard approach— even physical therapy—had been for me, I not only knew what to do, I relished the opportunity to make a difference in the lives of these suffering individuals, many of whom had already experienced every tragedy life can bring and struggled day-to-day just to survive.

I started a special group therapy to help these patients. And pursued other activities to make them better. I found that giving them activities that gave them control over their lives proved the most effective. In addition to daily exercise, meditation has proven beneficial. Group therapy proved to be a special setting for so many of these patients. It was not just me passing out wisdom and comfort. Insights and support came from many quarters.

Depression Proved a Major Blindspot

ONE DAY, I REALIZED the doctors sending depressed patients to me from the medical clinic were not making the connection between their patients' chronic pain and their depression, so I talked with the head of the medical clinic about the problems in the system. I gave talks to the staff, and he and I tried to work with other professionals at the hospital to address the chronic pain logjam since patients were being referred to the wrong clinics, clogging up the system.

Just when we were starting to make progress, the orthopedic doctor in charge of coordinating our activities left, and the administration turned over leadership to the anesthesiologist who gave spinal blocks for chronic pain in the pain clinic. This doctor did not see the need for dealing with depression or exercise, so he just dismissed the working group altogether!

Missing Depression and Suicidal Behavior

Over and over in my teaching activities and other interactions with doctors, depression stood out as a particular blind spot. This failure had devastating consequences in patients with chronic pain who may be given opiates or pain blocks under general anesthesia and never be assessed for depression, the underlying problem. Even exercise was seen as peripheral when dealing with depression and pain. In addition, suicidal patients were being missed completely.

One case of depression from one of the teaching conferences stands out in my mind: a patient on renal dialysis had become non-compliant with her doctor's instructions.

"What do you think that means?" I asked the student who presented the patient at our teaching conference.

"Non-compliance means the patient did not follow the doctor's instructions," the student responded.

"I'm not asking you what the word non-compliance means. I'm asking you what's going on with your patient that might cause her to ignore the doctor's instructions."

The student had no idea and had not even thought to find out. The patient in question was on permanent chronic dialysis. There was no kidney transplant in her future. She had stopped treatment as a way to end her life.

Depression should be evaluated and treated, especially in situations where the illness or the treatment can cause confusion. When any illness or treatment gives rise to depression, especially where the suicide rate is high, like dialysis, the suicide rate is up to 400 times the national average.

Non-compliance is the red flag, the warning sign. Failing to evaluate non-compliance, along with other behaviors and symptoms, limits the physician's ability to truly understand the patient and intervene when necessary. Depressed patients will neglect themselves. And while most medical patients won't put a gun to their heads to commit suicide, non-compliance amounts to the same thing.

In rounding with the medical team one morning, I found a diabetic who had stopped using insulin and a patient who would not give up smoking before her bypass surgery. The medical team relied on giving each patient a stern lecture rather than recognizing these behaviors as signs of depression and the suicide attempts they actually were.

The diabetic had already gone into a diabetic coma, which prompted the hospital admission. The bypass surgery would be canceled if the other patient continued to smoke. The medical team was shy about asking about suicidal thoughts as if they were suggesting suicide to the patient. But both talked readily about their suicidal thoughts when given a chance.

At the very least, the patient's ability to heal or even tolerate the pain and the indignity of medical treatment depends on having one's feelings understood. This fosters a necessary positive attitude toward the doctor and the medical team. A physician who is willing to ask hard questions and has the ability to understand contributes heavily to that bond.

Treating Chronic Pain Introduced Me to Alternative Therapies

AFTER I STARTED THE program focused on chronic pain, one of my friends, a yoga specialist, volunteered to do a guided meditation at the end of group. That proved most effective in teaching these patients how to relax and let go of the tension that worsened their pain.

As word got out about our program, some practitioners from the community volunteered to help. Some did massage therapy with our patients, and others volunteered to teach meditation. Exercise therapists from St. Vincent's Rehab Facility offered chair aerobics classes and let our patients come to swim classes in their pools.

Some local chiropractors were willing to come to the hospital to work with our patients, but the medical staff was leery. We could have had a specialist do acupuncture, but in Alabama, only a physician can do acupuncture in a hospital setting.

Starting the Endorphin Clinic

As part of assessing the need for a multi-disciplinary pain clinic at the hospital, I looked at opiate use in the various clinics. To my surprise, I found that what doctors prescribed had more to do with the doctor and his feelings about addiction and opiate use than it did with the patient's needs. Opiates were being handed out too freely by some doctors, while others refused to give any opiates at all.

Even when opiates were prescribed, they were not being used in the best way to help patients recover. They were not given to help patients do better, rather than just feel better. Rather than give opiates to help patients exercise or be more active, they were given for hurting. Improving function would further their chances of recovery from chronic pain. They were also not being taught how to avoid addiction or make their pain worse by not taking a regular dose.

I also found out the nurses knew of some patients who needed to sell their opiates for food or shelter, and other patients who were addicts targeting the medical clinics and the emergency rooms for opiates, causing problems for everyone.

Finally, after I asked the pharmacy to take a look at all opiate prescriptions in the hospital, the administration took note of the opiate problem in the hospital and turned to me to put together a multidisciplinary pain clinic to deal with chronic pain and depression, addicts with pain complaints, and referrals to specialty clinics like orthopedics, the pain block clinic, the rheumatology clinic, and others.

Our greatest challenge was getting doctors to change their traditional behavior and getting the nursing staff to see that giving an opiate prescription was not the clinic's primary function! I didn't recognize at the time how the focus on medication, to the exclusion of everything else, was an unconscious defense against anxiety.

How Chronic Pain Became the Vehicle for Understanding the Importance of Alternative Therapies

FINDING WAYS TO HELP this group of patients with a range of chronic pain issues introduced me to the myriad benefits of so-called alternative or natural therapies. From my own experience, I already knew the benefits of exercise to manage pain and depression. Since 80% of chronic pain is musculoskeletal, exercise and stretching are key to making a difference in most patients. Even in patients with other causes of pain, keeping the muscles, tendons, and fascia flexible is helpful. As I prepared for this clinic, I learned of more alternative treatments.

In the process of seeking the best program for our program, I talked with many practitioners around town and learned a lot about the treatment of pain in our community. I visited some clinics and talked with their staff. Some pain clinics just handed out medicines, mostly opiates. Others did only physical rehabilitation. Some did only massage therapy. Chiropractors did manipulations, nutrition counseling, and other procedures. Acupuncture clinics did their thing. And some general pain clinics offered a range of treatment options, including group therapy.

My sense was that those using opiates were giving too much since that's what kept patients coming back for more visits. A few clinic directors would not talk with me at all because they saw me as a competitor. However, one clinic owner was generous enough to let me come in one afternoon a week for six weeks so I could experience his clinic. He even offered to pay me, but I declined, feeling his time teaching me was worth far more. Through this mini-survey of what was available, I saw a great range of alternative therapies and opportunities for my patients.

More Alternative Therapies in Workshops

ONCE A QUARTER, THE social worker on our team organized a workshop to teach patients about pain and what they could do to improve. In the workshops, I learned more about alternative therapies, such as the effects of certain foods on the pain in certain individuals, as well as the beneficial effects of music therapy, various breathing rituals, meditation, nutritional therapy, and distraction to manage pain. Distraction is a major way of dealing with pain, whether it's through activity or focusing on the breath.

All these "alternative therapies" are skills we all can master to help us weather the inevitable pain and depression that life brings. Imagine the difference if we were all trained from childhood to incorporate exercise, stretching, deep breathing, music, meditation, and dietary change into our daily routines instead of being just taught, "If you hurt, take pills."

I called the Endorphin Clinic to emphasize we were encouraging activities that would release our own naturally occurring opiates, the endorphins, and to ensure patients did not have to keep hurting to participate in our activities. We had special groups for addicts and those with a sensitive nervous system who were more prone to migraines, TMJ, IBS, MVP, and those with chronic pain from inactivity or injury.

Making the System More Efficient

By having this clinic, we could triage all patients with chronic pain and get them to the right services. That way, the orthopedic clinic would not get referrals for those who did not need surgery, and patients needing surgery would not develop bad habits and chronic pain, waiting months just to get an appointment.

Also, since many pre- and post-surgery patients could not afford physical therapy, by including physical activity in our program, we could offset the need for expensive PT and avoid having patients just sit around developing chronic problems. We could also see that the exercise was focused on total body movement . . . not just focused on a small area.

When I started delving into the range of therapies relevant to chronic pain, I was surprised at how ignorant I was about so many alternative therapeutic activities that benefit those with chronic pain, as well as those with depression and anxiety.

Inspiring Change

MANY PATIENTS ARE HIGHLY reluctant to change anything in their lives. So, despite my stunning success with my first patient at the county hospital, my greatest challenge during the fifteen years I spent working with patients at Cooper Green was devising ways to inspire change. Seeing other patients alter their behavior and improve was a powerful motivator for some.

For many, finding a way to assert a little control over the uncertainty in their lives empowered tremendous change. So many patients lived in tremendously challenging circumstances, surrounded by poverty, violence, and ill health, that gaining some small element of control was huge. The two most successful items I had to offer in this regard proved to be exercise and meditation.

Already familiar with the benefits of exercise, I encouraged patients to start doing what they could. If they were terribly out of shape, I encouraged walking just a little four times a day. If they could only walk to the bathroom, I encouraged them to walk back and forth twice each time they went. If they could not walk, I showed them how to exercise in a chair and, if possible, put on music and dance where they were—even in bed.

Once that activity became routine, they could gradually increase their weekly activity. Even patients with severe respiratory and cardiac problems were able to do a little more in time and found it helped their breathing and pain.

The Magic of Meditation

MEDITATION WAS THE FIRST alternative therapy I learned about in the clinic. Several people volunteered to do meditation workshops with our patients. In addition, I learned to do guided meditations after my group therapy sessions so patients would leave feeling relaxed and would see the effect of meditating on their pain levels.

I already knew about the benefits of progressive relaxation techniques and biofeedback in training patients to relax in my private practice, but even without the tapes or biofeedback equipment, I was stunned by the power of meditation to alter lives.

Those doing daily meditation at home talked about how it made them more aware of everything in their lives: their relationships, anger, and even their relationship with food. I encouraged patients to experiment with their own guided meditations and notice when meditation techniques worked best for them. Some were very creative and devised their own messages to focus on. Others incorporated meditation into their morning exercise routine.

The most dramatic effect of meditation occurred in a disheveled homeless woman sent to me for depression and pain in her arm. She kept hitting out with her arm, even though it hurt.

"I can't do this breathing exercise," she complained one day after my guided meditation.

I'd noticed her getting increasingly agitated as I went through the routine, even though I tried to tie it to our previous discussion. "Just think about what was said today," I said. "Think about how angry you are with your brother for not protecting you from getting raped."

She looked at me. "Is that why I keep hitting out?" she asked. "Just like how I want to punch him in the nose?"

I nodded. This woman had been in and out of jail and psychiatric hospitals for years for "losing it" on the street. Perhaps her pain and hitting gestures were an unconscious way for her to protect herself from being locked up again.

As was so often the case with patients at the county hospital, I did not see this woman again for six months. When she finally came back, she was beaming.

"I'm never going to jail again," she boasted. "The next time I get mad, I'm just going to do my breathing exercises and let it go!"

Those of us who grew up in privileged circumstances forget how too many neglected kids do not get the training they need in childhood to handle their emotions in order to survive comfortably in this world. This woman, who had never gotten past the third grade, quickly learned skills that could help her survive.

One day, after the clinic had been running for several months, I got a call from a friend of a friend who wanted me to see his sister, who had been to every doctor in town and many out of town for treatment of her pain. She had recently returned from a month-long program and was worse than ever.

Inwardly, I groaned. What could I do in my little Jerry-rigged clinic to make a difference? "She'll have to come to Cooper Green and register," I said. "And be sure she sends us all her records."

One day, without being seen by me and the rest of the team, she was in a group with all the other patients. I introduced myself, as I always did, and encouraged her to do the same when it was her turn.

I had long since gotten over wondering what I would do with too many patients in the room. Those who were relatively stable seemed to recognize who was in trouble and needed to talk, so although everyone got to introduce themselves and talk as I went around the circle, I never knew who or what would be the group's focus that day. That meant the new patient had been coming to group hearing from many people for several weeks before I ever saw her with her records.

To my amazement, she picked up on the daily exercise and meditation and started to improve even before I had a chance to see her and make recommendations. In the end, she needed to be weaned off her medications, which were making her hurt more, but it was clear she was empowered to take steps on her own by coming to group and hearing the stories of others.

The ultimate lesson was helping patients develop a routine that worked for them in their lives. Since we all are different, having a routine that addresses each person's situation was key. If it was not a routine, the improvement would not last, and they would be right back where they had been before. Perhaps that is why the patient who just came to group did so well. She was developing her own routine.

This experience piqued my interest in learning more about alternative treatment approaches. I found some had been around for hundreds of years, while others were developed in response to a void in what medicine had to offer.

*"Our food should be our medicine and our
medicine should be our food."*
— HIPPOCRATES

*"It is easier to change a man's religion
than to change his diet."*
— MARGARET MEAD

*"The doctor of the future will no longer treat the
human frame with drugs, but rather will cure
and prevent disease with nutrition."*
— THOMAS A. EDISON

*"I got into being vegan because I was simply looking to
benefit from being more compassionate. I have since come
to learn that it is an animal-based diet that is responsible
for the overwhelming majority of cases of cancer,
heart disease, diabetes, obesity, multiple sclerosis,
and all kinds of other problems."*
— STEVE-O

"Optimum nutrition is the medicine of tomorrow."
— LINUS PAULING

CHAPTER THIRTEEN

So, What About Food?

In 1994, after my daughter finished graduate school at the University of Michigan, I traveled with her to São Paulo, Brazil, to visit her violin teacher, who had moved back home after several years in the U.S.

Due to the crush of homeless people all over Brazil and the violence everywhere on the streets in São Paulo, it was no longer safe for women to go outside by themselves, even in the daytime. Everyone in São Paulo lived behind walls; the richer you were, the grander your wall. Cars were parked in garages, not on the street. So, when the music teacher gave violin lessons in her living room, I had to read in the bedroom.

One of the books I found on her bookshelf was Jean Carper's *Food: Your Miracle Medicine*. This book outlined the importance of what we put in our mouths to prevent and reverse heart disease, cancer, and other diseases. Why, I wondered, have I, as a physician, not heard this before? I was stunned. I had been a physician for about twenty-five years, but everything in this book was new to me.

Always investigating new ideas, I considered myself well-versed in the subject of nutrition. I even developed an educational simulation related to eating behavior called Binge Buster. This educational game emphasized that foods in the U.S. are made to sell, not to make us healthy. I demonstrated how preservatives are made to extend the food's shelf life, not to extend consumers' lives. I had even included facts like "sugar and salt are added to many foods to make them more irresistible, not more nutritious."

Somewhere along the way, I had read about the Norwegians whose health improved during WWII after the Nazi Germans confiscated all their animals. The incidence of cancer and heart disease went down. After the war, when the Norwegians got their herds back, their higher rates of cancer and heart disease returned to pre-war levels.

In addition, I had read about foreigners from countries with a lower incidence of heart disease coming to the U.S. and developing the same incidence of heart disease as Americans after eating our diet. But still, that did not convince me enough to give up eating meat.

I even knew firsthand the unwise practice of eating the wrong foods. At a medical meeting in Atlanta before boarding the plane to São Paulo, I had eaten too many salty peanuts, and my legs were massively swollen when our plane got to Brazil. By eating lots of fruits—many I had never heard of before—like guarana and putting my feet up on a wall for several hours a day, my return home was easy, and I had no problem with swelling.

Still, after reading Carper's book, I was not persuaded enough to change my diet completely after I got home. I did make sure I ate nine fruits and vegetables every day, though. I thought maybe vegetables would help me cut down on the bad things in my diet.

I did not realize then how addicted I was to certain foods, sweets in particular. I still wondered why my ice cream craving seemed worse after having a big meal and dessert. Despite working with drug addicts, I did not see what I had to do to solve my problem.

Then, after the start of the Endorphin clinic in 2003, at one of our workshops on managing pain, I learned how foods can actually increase or cause pain in susceptible individuals. In the part of that workshop focused on food, a nutritionist showed how, in addition to the stress from too much weight on our joints from obesity, eating certain foods made arthritis and other pains worse.

She talked about one man who could not eat red meat because it made his arthritis flare. Another could not eat nightshade vegetables[24] because of pain, the significant factor here was inflammation. Apparently, certain foods encourage inflammation, which makes pain worse. Foods causing inflammation, it seems, include alcohol, sugar, certain grains, dairy products, red meat, and processed foods.[25]

Caffeine may cause pain through increased acidity or may cause pain in the withdrawal phase as the effects of the caffeine wear off. If you have gout, canned fish—like herring, sardines, and anchovies—may increase your pain. Each person must be aware of what foods may increase pain or cause other problems.

I was using exercise and stretching to manage chronic pain, so I had not even considered that food might have that effect on me as well until I realized that my early morning headaches might be withdrawal from caffeine.

Fat, Sick, and Nearly Dead

THEN, IN 2012, I ran across the documentary *Fat, Sick and Nearly*

24 Nightshade vegetables: tomatoes, eggplant, potatoes, and peppers.

25 Processed foods include anything which is not a natural substance: many items we buy in the market and have when we eat fast food.

Dead. In the movie, a young man from Australia, weighing close to 400 pounds, starts juicing for all his meals to lose weight and correct his medical problems: diabetes, hypertension, and heart disease caused by what he ate.

In the movie, the young man drives around the U.S., juicing as he goes. He juices his fruits and vegetables right out of the back of his car, encouraging other overweight people along the way to juice with him. As he and the others in the movie lose weight, they are able to get off medications for diabetes, hypertension, and heart disease bit by bit.

That movie showed how juicing can not only correct obesity but also reverse life-threatening health conditions caused by eating the wrong diet. In this movie, eating fruits and vegetables, in this instance in the form of juice, got people off medications by reversing serious health conditions like diabetes, hypertension, and heart disease.

After that, my husband and I started juicing one day a week and really looked at what we ate. At the same time, I was researching the effects of diet on pain for my second book,[26] a self-help book about chronic pain, depression, and addiction.

That's when I found T. Colin Campbell's book, *The China Study.* In this book, Dr. Campbell describes his efforts to share his research about the dangers of the American diet with the public, only to find he was unable to get the government to act on the science because members of the food industry run the government agencies overseeing food recommendations to the public. That's when he decided to write the book.

In the book, he describes how two research studies showed him

26   *HEAL: What You Can Do to Treat Chronic Pain, Depression and Addiction.*

how our meat diet was causing us to get cancer. In one study, he looked at people in Asia who got their protein from plants, and his other study looked at a cancer population of Americans. Seeing the low incidence of cancer in his Asian subjects made him curious about the effects of diet on the incidence of cancer.

I also discovered Caldwell Esselstyn's book, *How to Prevent and Reverse Heart Disease*. It appears one can reverse the damaging effects of the American diet by eating a different way. After that, there was an explosion of books, TV programs, videos, and internet events talking about the dangers of the American diet, the role of the GI tract in the immune system, and the role of diet in feeding the healthy bacteria in the gut or, alternatively, feeding the gut dangerous bacteria with the wrong diet: the standard American diet.

Many people in America started shifting away from the standard fare to embrace grass-fed meat, free-range chickens, and diets free of gluten, salt, sugar, and processed foods. Kale suddenly became popular.

As I learned about food and the American way of eating, I tried to make lasting changes to my diet, to eat more of an anti-inflammatory diet: fruits, vegetables, and whole grains. I eliminated sugar, wheat, dairy, and processed foods. Unfortunately, over and over again, I found it too easy to slip back into old habits.

Heart Doctors Use Stents Rather Than Talk About Diet

THEN, IN 2013, MY husband went in for hip surgery. During the procedure, his EKG revealed some heart problems. The staff rushed him to cardiac catheterization, where they put two little mesh tubes called stents in his narrowed vessels and, even though he was not having chest pain, put him on a blood thinner, Plavix plus Statins.

My husband had a regular exercise routine three times a week at the rehab center where I went to swim, but he also rushed to sign up for the cardiac rehab program of monitored exercise.

Throughout this whole episode, no one mentioned diet to him. At no time did a doctor ask my husband, "What do you eat?" Or say, "Here is a book you need to read about reversing heart disease. We now know you can reverse cardiac problems through what you eat." In fact, the cardiologist never recommended anything on the subject.

A year later, he was quick to order another cardiac catheterization to see the stents, which by then had collapsed.

My husband was very active, playing tennis, boating, and working in the yard. On Plavix, the blood-thinner medication, he bled profusely every time he got a small cut. One day, he slipped in his boat and was covered in blood. I could not help but think, "What if he had hit his head!"

After that, my frustration with his doctor reached a boiling point, and I called a cardiologist friend of mine. By then, I had read that Plavix led to more bleeds in the brain than initially expected. I wanted my husband off Plavix and to see a different doctor.

I wanted someone who would address food, not just perform potentially hazardous procedures. When we got the new doctor, even he did not think you could reverse heart disease that was already there. He did eat a healthy diet himself to avoid getting heart disease, but thought my husband must have permanent damage.

Later my husband got stage 4 kidney disease. Why, I thought didn't his doctors get him to alter his diet before he got to this point. Much is known about protecting the kidney by what we eat, but none of his doctors seemed to be aware of that. All they knew had to do with talking medicines….which had side effects that made him worse.

Then, in 2019, I was admitted to the hospital with sepsis. I did well enough initially because I was not seriously ill. However, I was sick for months after leaving the hospital. The antibiotics had wiped out the bugs in my GI tract, and needless to say, I made it worse by what I ate: an inflammatory diet.

In the hospital, the food was a horror show. It represented the very worst of the American diet: lots of fat, salt, and processed foods. It certainly was not an anti-inflammatory diet (fruits, vegetables, whole grains, beans, nuts, and no processed foods), which might have helped my immune system fight off the infection and trained me how to eat once I went home in order to grow a healthy microbiome.[27]

What a lost opportunity to teach me and other patients how best to eat to facilitate recovery and, for some patients, to reverse conditions like chronic pain, diabetes, heart disease, dementia, and cancer.

I did not get better until nearly Christmas when I took a probiotic to replenish the bacteria in my gut and gave up eating sweets.

Treating MS and Other Chronic Illness

FAILURE TO CONSIDER NATURAL therapies like diet and exercise can be very costly for those with chronic illnesses like multiple sclerosis. No neurologist has ever asked me about exercise or stretching. They have never taken a history of my exercise routine. Nor has anyone made the connection between antibiotic use, which tends to make me weaker and bring out old MS symptoms, and the status of my GI tract and my immune system. My doctors have not zeroed in on what I have been eating, which may have contributed to my having more infections and kept me from exercising as much as I should.

By getting patients to focus on a diet solely for weight loss and not on the role of food in managing health and disease, doctors do

---

27   Microbiome involves all the collection of all microbes, such as bacteria, fungi, viruses, and their genes, that naturally live inside and on us and interact with our nervous system in various ways.

a real disservice to their patients. Excess weight and the food that results in excess weight cause an increase in chronic inflammation that can give rise to gout, diabetes, heart disease, and cancer.

But doctors don't even need to manage the patient's diet; they could just refer them to a dietitian or a book on nutrition to help them acquire health. They could even give patients a pamphlet about diet and exercise as religiously as they do a pamphlet about the privacy of information. Getting doctors to focus on insurance and filling out forms has shifted their focus away from finding what is best for their patients.

Why Chronic Inflammation Matters—What Diet Can Do

ACUTE INFLAMMATION MAY BE brought on by infectious agents like bacteria and viruses or non-infectious events like injuries, poisons, or stress. In contrast, chronic inflammation is a long-term physiological response that can last from weeks to years.

Unlike acute inflammation, chronic inflammation is not always visible to the naked eye. It can be brought on by a number of factors, including autoimmune conditions, chronic stress, long-term exposure to pollutants, physical inactivity, or foods and drinks we routinely consume. A state of constant inflammatory response can create chains of destructive bodily reactions that damage cells and are linked to conditions like chronic pain, gout, diabetes, cardiovascular disease, dementia, depression, and even cancers.

A Diet to Treat Pain

AS WE LOOK MORE and more at the bacteria that live with us and interact with our nervous system, the food we eat every day and the drinks we reach for to quench our thirst matter more and more. Ancient skeletons don't show signs of arthritis, so something about our modern diet is making us sick and causing us to have more and more health problems.[28]

Food is an important ingredient in living a life pain-free. Pursuing an anti-inflammatory diet[29] gives us the best chance of not having pain triggered by what we eat. The anti-inflammatory diet discussed at length by Dr. Joel Fuhrman[30] is one example. More and more, the internet has a lot of recommendations about anti-inflammatory foods.

The irony here is that if we give up eating too much salt, sugar, and fat, our taste buds change within two weeks. After a very short time, food starts tasting too salty. Sweets taste excessively rich and cloying, like cotton candy.

Beyond that, once our taste buds are not sullied by artificial sugar and white flour, natural foods taste sweeter with an amazing range of subtle flavors previously drowned out by the sugar. We get to enjoy the benefit of natural flavors. Carrots become amazingly sweet; other fruits and vegetables reveal their flavor treasures.

Sadly, because doctors are so specialized these days, too often, they do not address a range of issues that make and keep patients well. Physicians need to address what patients eat and how they exercise during any illness and every recovery period. To dismiss these interventions as lifestyle issues is to miss an opportunity to get patients healthy again during an infection and after it is gone.

My regular doctor never saw me at all when I went to the hospital

---

28 B. Brett Finlay & Jessica M. Finlay, *The Whole-Body Microbiome: How to Harness Microbes Inside and Out for Lifelong Health.*

29 Anti-inflammatory diet consists of no sugar, no dairy, no wheat, and no processed food at least 80% of the time.

30 Dr. Joel Fuhrman, *The Anti-Inflammatory Diet.*

with a blood infection. The hospitalist doctor who treated my sepsis in the hospital never saw me again, so where was I to learn about what to eat and how to exercise during my recovery?

With what we now know about diet, it should be malpractice not to discuss the role of diet in recovery from infections, heart disease, cancer, or other conditions with patients in the hospital. The hospital food service could be the first place to begin the education. The medical society should take the lead and even fine doctors who fail to address these important issues.

Foods That Fight Inflammation

Special foods that fight inflammation include those with polyphenols such as onions, turmeric, red grapes, tart cherries, plums, blueberries, pumpkin seeds, salmon, chili peppers, leafy vegetables like spinach, kale, and collards, coffee, cocoa, green tea, plus extra virgin olive oil for omega-3 oils, ginger[31] and bananas.[32]

Foods That Cause Inflammation or Make It Worse

SOME OF THE WORST foods for inflammation include refined carbohydrates with sugar and white flour, processed meats, red meat, baked goods, sweetened beverages, trans fat, and omega-6 fatty acids like corn oil, sunflower oil, and vegetable oil—plus processed foods. And, for some, nightshade vegetables.

---

31   A staple of traditional medicine, this pungent root is probably best known for its anti-nausea, stomach-soothing properties.

32   Eaten during exercise bananas are equal to sports drinks. They contain metabolites that function like ibuprofen.

"Homeopathy...cures a larger percentage of cases than any other method of treatment and is beyond doubt safer and more economical than most complete science."
— MAHATMA GHANDI

"You may honestly feel grateful that homeopathy survived the attempts of the allopaths (orthodoxy) to destroy it."
— MARK TWAIN

Understanding How Homeopathy and Other Natural or Alternative Medical Therapies Became Discredited

My education in medicine was very traditional, and I always saw myself as a traditional medical practitioner, making diagnoses and plugging in the proper medication. As a psychiatrist, I also saw my role as understanding what was troubling the patient and working to resolve their issues.

In the 1960s, when I first went into medicine, we had no training to consider exercise or diet as natural therapies. Natural therapies like homeopathy were considered ineffectual. I remember hearing, "The dosages they use in homeopathy are too small to be of any use."

Then, about twenty years ago, I heard homeopathy treatments were found to have a placebo effect. Around the same time, I also learned that the history of medical treatment is essentially the history of the placebo effect. In other words, all treatments have a placebo effect.

Placebo, that mysterious, oft-misunderstood force that encourages us to get well and is used routinely as the standard against every new drug or treatment, must be tested: the double-blind controlled trial.

Many traditional therapies, used for thousands of years, have been found to promote healing, presumably through the placebo effect. In addition to boosting the immune system, some traditional therapies encourage more activity and better eating and sleeping habits. In other words, they encourage people to act well, which is ultimately needed to get well.

In my early days in medicine, we kept patients in bed too long, recovering from surgeries or heart attacks. My grandmother stayed flat on her back for three months following a hip replacement in 1978. Now, we try to get people moving as soon as possible for a faster recovery. We even give strong opiates after surgery, so patients will start moving around sooner. Patients need to move and act well to get well.

Being introduced to alternative approaches to chronic pain at the county hospital, Cooper Green, led me to read about homeopathy and other alternative therapies. What a surprise that turned out to be.

Homeopathy is a medical system based on the belief that the body can cure itself given the proper support from the environment. Developed in Germany in 1796 by Dr. Samuel Hahnemann, homeopathic medicines use tiny amounts of natural substances, like plants and minerals, in their medicines. Dr. Hahnemann believed these medicines stimulate the healing process.

Dr. Hahnemann was an impressive figure. A graduate of two medical schools, he spoke and read seven languages, so he had reviewed medical treatments worldwide. He opposed the standard treatment of his time, which was still based on the four humors. This prevailing approach was toxic and frequently made patients worse.

Instead, Hahnemann developed a type of treatment that was safe to use as well as effective in helping his patients get well. As a physician who has recognized many limitations in my own profession, I could identify with the frustration this highly trained and knowledgeable physician must have had with his profession.

Dr. Hahnemann first used the word "allopath" in 1810 as a derogatory term for practitioners of so-called "heroic medicine," the traditional medicine in Europe at the time and the predecessor to today's standard medicine in the U.S. and Europe.

Heroic medicine was based on the belief that disease is caused by an imbalance among the four "humors," blood, phlegm, yellow bile, and black bile. This belief originated with Hippocrates and Galen before the birth of Christ. Heroic medicine sought to treat disease symptoms by correcting humoral imbalances using harsh and abusive methods like bleeding, purging, enemas, and toxic chemicals to induce symptoms seen as the opposite of those produced by specific diseases.

Even in the 19th century, the medicines they used contained mercury, lead, and arsenic. This form of medical treatment is credited with maiming or killing many. Perhaps the poor were lucky they couldn't afford to see a doctor when they got sick!

Recognizing the Benefits of Homeopathy

DURING THE CHOLERA OUTBREAK in London in 1854, many people died. Epidemiology got its start when Dr. John Snow tracked the outbreak back to one specific water source in London.

After the disease had receded, the medical establishment, which consisted of allopathic doctors, performed a study of the most effective cholera treatments. They found the death rate at the hospital using standard allopathic treatment methods, such as bleeding, purging, enemas, and toxic chemicals listed above, was 50 percent, about the same as the untreated death rate.

However, the death rate at the homeopathic hospital using standard homeopathic methods, given the proper support from the environment, was a fraction of that—just 16.4%.

Homeopathic hospitals were more focused on making the patients comfortable, replacing fluids, and giving medicine to facilitate their own recovery from disease rather than giving treatments that would worsen dehydration and stress vulnerable patients.

The results were so shocking that the allopathic doctors refused to include the homeopathy results in their report. They went further, trying to suggest the homeopathic hospital was not even treating cholera patients or was only treating milder cases, even though the allopathic doctors' own investigator had reported otherwise. This is only one blatant example of allopathic doctors trying to discredit homeopathy, a natural therapy, which represented competition with their own treatments.[33]

Today, various homeopathic methods and medicines are still used to prevent and treat outbreaks of cholera around the world, most notably in Africa. We now know cholera does not have to be lethal if fluids are replaced as they are being lost to diarrhea and vomiting. So, homeopathic methods have found a place in cholera treatment around the world today.[34]

33   Dean ME, "Selective Suppression by the medical establishment of unwelcome research findings: The cholera treatment evaluation by the General Board of Health," London, 1854, 2020: JLL Bulletin Commentaries on the history of treatment evaluation.

34   "History: The Homeopathic Treatment and Prevention of Cholera (Part B),"

Allopathic Medicine Co-opts American Medicine

DID YOU KNOW OUR current medical system was not always the only one, with everything else considered secondary? In 1844, the American Institute of Homeopathy was formed as America's first national medical society. Alarmed, allopathic doctors formed the American Medical Association (AMA) in 1846.

Despite some success, the AMA was a weak organization with little money or respect among the general public until George H. Simmons took charge of it in 1899. Under Dr. Simmons's direction, the AMA pursued multiple avenues to gain control over the practice of medicine and profit monetarily from that power.

Big Pharma's Takeover of Medicine

PATENT MEDICINES WERE FIRST described and advertised in the 18th century. The Food and Drug Administration (FDA) was formed in the U.S. in 1906 to assess and regulate the veracity of claims about drugs and prescription medicines. Ironically, it was not until the onset of modern TV commercials for drugs, starting in 1997, that drug advertising became widespread and unregulated.

The practice of marketing medical services, hospitals, and medical practices, in addition to prescription drugs, skyrocketed between 1997 and 2016, contributing to a massive rise in medical fees and the outrageous costs of prescription drugs we see today. Today, medicine has become a for-profit organization owned for the most part by big business and not an enterprise to address the nation's health.

High-tech medicine is the best in the world, with advances in surgery, anesthesia, gene therapy, and more. But so much of that

Internet for discussion of specific remedies.

treatment is out of bounds for those who don't have the money, and in other areas, general approaches to healthcare lag behind.

As a young physician, I was aware of the prohibition against advertising in medicine. I assumed these were ethical norms for the profession of medicine. While taking a course in public health, I learned about the strong prohibition in this country against "restraint of trade"—that is, making money takes a higher priority than other values in a court of law, so making money has a higher priority than ethical norms.

Before 1997, advertising in medicine was considered unethical since ads appeal to emotions and don't present the full picture of risk, benefit, and cost that doctors must weigh before treating their patients. But in 1997, the FDA approved letting drug companies advertise their products on TV. That opened the floodgates to all kinds of advertising of medical practices, individual doctors, and medical centers.

When I searched for an explanation as to why the United States alone, apart from New Zealand, permits such activity, I discovered the dark history of American medicine's takeover by allopathic medicine, which goes back more than a hundred years. This exposes a dark side of the profession I have labored in most of my life. I was shocked.

Even worse, no physician I talked to after learning this history had ever heard about it. Some had even spent their professional lives carving out academic successes based on testing drugs in placebo-controlled trials at many universities.

"*The art of medicine consists in amusing the patient while nature cures the disease.*"
— Voltaire

"*Human history becomes more and more a race between education and catastrophe.*"
— H.G. Wells (1866-1946), historian and science fiction writer, "The Fate of Homo Sapiens," p. 105, 1920

"*I think modern medicine has become like a prophet offering a life free of pain. It is nonsense. The only thing I know that truly heals people is unconditional love.*"
— Elisabeth Kubler-Ross

CHAPTER FIFTEEN

History Of Medicine's War on Natural Therapies

Medicine's war on natural therapies goes back centuries. From the beginning of time, women have traditionally been responsible for nurturing the sick, the wounded, the young, the pregnant, the old, and the dying. Theirs was the caring role, the consistent day-to-day involvement with health. Their interventions encouraged progress and mitigated the consequences of illness or injury.

Women often relied on remedies passed down through their families and local traditions. Some were exceptionally gifted healers who helped others in trouble. They were often involved in treating women's health issues and delivering babies.

As early as the 1300s, priests and male doctors began organized efforts to destroy women healers. Ravaged by war, overcrowding, unsanitary conditions, and massive crop failures, Europe was ripe for the plague and other diseases that swept across the continent.

Just as the church demonized women as being responsible for adultery, it also demonized women healers as the cause of other problems, including natural disasters, male impotency, crop failures, abnormal births, the death of farm animals, and diseases male doctors could not heal.

To treat illnesses during the Middle Ages and up through the 19th century, male doctors applied leeches, employed bloodletting, conducted horrific surgeries without anesthesia, and prescribed various chemicals, many of them toxic. Most of the actual care of the sick was undertaken by women healers who used herbs and traditional remedies.

Many of these unlicensed healers were accused of being witches. Most often, it was widows, women who had never married, and poor women who were thus accused.

From the 14th to the 17th century, *thousands* of women were killed, often by being burned at the stake by Catholic and Protestant churches. These gruesome executions were public events in which the victims were often tortured before they were killed.

In England, the belief that witches could do supernatural harm to others by using spells, medicines, or charms led to the passage of three different Witchcraft Acts in 1542, 1563, and 1604. Even after the laws were repealed, village people continued to believe in witches and conduct violence against them.

Although I'd heard about the burning of witches and other undesirable people like the mentally ill, I did not connect the destruction of witches to the threat male doctors felt from women healers, nor to the success of the witch hunts in wiping out women healers and excluding women from the study of medicine.

In Europe, women's healing role was not always appreciated by the church or the medical profession, both of which have long been run by men. The Middle Ages saw unprecedented violence against women healers. Women who had been called physicians in the 13th century were considered charlatans in the

14th and 15th centuries. Some of the antagonism against women was financial. Men did not want the competition, but after the plague swept through Europe, many of these women healers were made scapegoats and burned at the stake as witches by the Catholic and Lutheran churches.

Just as we hear about conspiracy theories affecting many today, the churches of the Middle Ages were just as affected by their fear that, through the plague and other diseases, God was wreaking vengeance on mankind for his sinful ways. While statues of naked women were destroyed and grand churches were built in their stead, more than 100,000 women were burned at the stake over several centuries.

Attacks on midwiferies were especially virulent. If the baby did not survive or if the mother died, the midwife was often accused of being in league with the devil. Malleus Maleficarum, or Hammer of Witches (1486), remained the official church text on witch hunting for three hundred years. This text claimed there were perverse sexual practices between witches and the devil.

While some European women could practice medicine, various attempts to exclude women from the profession continued throughout the Middle Ages. With the rise of universities, women were refused entrance, creating a legal male monopoly on the practice of medicine. Women claimed this unfair discrimination occurred because they were seen as competing with the men who practiced medicine.

To this day, the war against women in education, medicine, and other professions—and even against allowing women to have control over their own bodies and health—continues.

In the summer of 2022, the U.S. Supreme Court overruled Roe v. Wade, ending a woman's forty-year right to have control over her own health and body. In our enlightened age, the courts and the medical profession seem to be still at war with women and natural therapies that have healed people for generations.[35]

How American Medical Activities Get Into the Battle

TO UNDERSTAND HOW MEDICAL practice became so alienated from natural therapies and the placebo effect, it's good to look at what medicine was like in the 19th century. American medical schools began opening in the late 18th century, but many doctors still trained in Europe. The body was generally thought to heal itself, so many healers called themselves "doctor" without any formal training.[36]

Women's health issues were mostly dealt with by other women. If a woman stopped having her period, it was assumed she was pregnant. Many women did not want to carry a child for various reasons, such as lack of food to feed the child, rape, etc.

To some, a lack of periods meant the body was out of balance and needed to be remedied. Abortion was widely accepted, except within some churches, which made contraception of any kind forbidden. Many women commonly took so-called "emmenagogues," drugs designed to stimulate menstrual flow, or used herbal remedies and folk practices like hot bricks on the abdomen to bring on periods.

If this did not work, a woman could buy patent medicines like Sir James Clarke's "female pills," which contained oil of say, or use mifepristone and misoprostol to restore female regularity. If that did not work, they could see a woman doctor specializing in female health issues, contraception, and abortion. Many of these women "doctors" had no formal training.

---

35   Wiliam L. Minkowski, MD, MPH, "Women Healers of the Middle Ages: Selected Aspects of Their History," AmJPublic Health, 1992, 82: 288-295.

36   Bettmann Archive/Getty Images.

One such woman, Ann Lohman, ended countless pregnancies during her forty-year career as Madame Restell. Although not officially trained, Lohman made a career of selling patent medicines and helping pregnant women who did not wish to give birth for fear of losing their reputations. Lohman's business was so well-known—and so successful—that it inspired copycats and helped create a booming abortion business in American cities.

By the mid-19th century, the practice of medicine was becoming an actual profession instead of just a group of homegrown practitioners. This led to the rise of more medical schools and accreditation, creating a class of professional doctors, largely men. About half of these professionals were trained in homeopathic medical colleges and half in allopathic medical schools.

Physicians coming out of both types of medical schools were suspicious of the midwives and the self-styled "doctors" many women relied on for abortions. As soon as the "allopaths" formed the American Medical Association (AMA) in 1847, its members began agitating to make abortion illegal. To do so, they challenged the common perception that a fetus was not a person until the pregnant mother felt it "quicken" or move. Even churches made a distinction between women who terminated their pregnancies pre- or post-quickening.

Before this time, abortion and the use of chemicals to end pregnancy were widely accepted and even advertised in the newspapers. That changed when the AMA targeted the midwives and others responsible for the care of women's health in order to capture the field of obstetrics and gynecology for male doctors.

The AMA's efforts were led by Horatio Storer, an obstetrician often called the father of American gynecology. Storer did not want the medical profession to be associated with abortion and considered a woman's desire to terminate her pregnancy tantamount to insanity.

He believed that a woman's biological role was to be a wife and mother and that to disrupt that path was not just to commit a social crime but murder. The AMA pushed for state laws to restrict abortions, and most states enacted them by 1880. The Comstock Law, passed by Congress in 1873, banned the sale of abortion drugs.

Let us not forget this was prior to the advent of antibiotics and vaccines, when many children did not survive to adulthood. This was brought home to me in 1988, sitting in a cemetery in northern England to watch the sunset. I could not help but notice a headstone nearby from less than one hundred years before. A man and his wife had had nine children. Only one lived to adulthood, and that child died at age 32.

Since then, sanitation, antibiotics, and vaccines have saved the lives of many adults and children, affecting how many children a woman needs to produce to have a family.

"*The person who takes medicine must recover twice, once from the disease and once from the medicine.*"
— WILLIAM OSLER

"*Be careful about reading health books. You may die of a misprint.*"
— MARK TWAIN

CHAPTER SIXTEEN

American Medical Association Enters the Medical Drama

A merica's first national medical society was formed in 1844: the American Institute of Homeopathy. Alarmed, allopathic doctors formed the American Medical Association (AMA) in 1846. From its inception, the AMA was involved in questionable activities and practices.[37]

Dr. George H. Simmons and Dr. Morris Fishbein established the AMA Council on Medical Education, which certified medical schools. To do this, the AMA developed guidelines that automatically gave lower ratings to homeopathic colleges, including those at Boston University and the University of Michigan, as well as New York Homeopathic Medical College and Hahnemann Medical College of Philadelphia.

---

37 Dana Ullman, MPH, CCH, adapted from an excerpt of *The Homeopathic Revolution: Why Famous People and Cultural Heroes Choose Homeopathy*, Berkeley: North Atlantic Books, 2007. How the AMA Got Rich & Powerful: "The AMA's Seal of Approval" George H. Simmons came up with the brilliant idea to transform the AMA into a big business by granting the AMA's "seal of approval" to certain drug companies that placed large and frequent ads in JAMA and its various affiliate publications.

This happened when twice as many students from homeopathic medical schools passed the medical boards as students from allopathic medical schools. This competition eventually led to the end of homeopathic medical schools altogether.

Morris Fishbein was a physician and editor of the Journal of the American Medical Association from 1924 to 1950. There are numerous stories about Fishbein's efforts to purchase the rights to various healing treatments.

Whenever the owner refused to sell such rights, Fishbein would label the treatment quackery.[38] If the owner of the treatment or device was a doctor, Fishbein would attack this doctor in his writings and place him on the AMA's "quackery list."

If the owner was not a doctor, it was common for them to be arrested for practicing medicine without a license or have their product confiscated by the Food and Drug Administration (FDA) or the Federal Trade Commission (FTC). Fishbein denied these allegations, but the AMA was tried and convicted of antitrust violations for conspiracy and restraint of trade in 1937. Fishbein also wrote health guides not based on scientific evidence.

In addition, Simmons set up the AMA's "Seal of Approval" to force drug companies to pay for ads in *The Journal of the American Medical Association* (JAMA). A drug company did not have to conduct any research or prove the safety or efficacy of a drug. All they had to do to gain approval was advertise in JAMA.[39]

---

38   Ausubel, 2000.

39   Dana Ullman, MPH, CCH, Contributor, *Evidence-Based Homeopath.* How the AMA Got Rich & Powerful: "The AMA's Seal of Approval" George H. Simmons came up with the brilliant idea to transform the AMA into a big business by granting the AMA's "seal of approval" to certain drug companies that placed large and frequent ads in JAMA and its various affiliate publications.

In 1913, Dr. Simmons and the AMA went on the offensive by establishing the organization's "Propaganda Department," dedicated explicitly to attacking any and all unconventional medical treatments and anyone (MD or not) who practiced them.

Simmons was later driven out of the AMA, but his model for extracting fees for branding medical practices and products persisted. Simmons's focus on molding public opinion also became one of the greatest weapons of the AMA, expanding to communicate the AMA's views through a syndicated column published in over 200 newspapers, a weekly radio program, and various books about how homeopathic practices and non-AMA-approved drugs were "quackery."[40] Still, the AMA was ineffective at discrediting homeopathy until J.D. Rockefeller entered the picture.

---

40   "Chiropractors sue AMA for antitrust - Wilk v. American Medical Association," 895: F.2d 352, 7th Cir. 1990.

"*It is not the strongest of the species that survives, nor the most intelligent, but the one most responsive to change.*"
— CHARLES DARWIN

"*Why do they call it 'Alternative Medicine' when it is the 'original medicine' humans have been using for over thousands of years? Chemical medications were only discovered about one hundred years ago.*"
— JON KABOT ZIN

Rockefeller Medicine: How the Actions of One Man Changed the Direction of Medicine in America

John D. Rockefeller was born on July 8, 1839. During his lifetime, natural therapies were very popular with the public. Homeopathy was only one of many widespread natural therapies, and even Rockefeller enjoyed the benefits of homeopathy.

In 1900, at least half the medical schools in the United States were based on natural therapies. The allopathic medical schools were the ones teaching surgery and the use of leeches and toxic substances such as mercury to treat cancer and other diseases, but they also taught some natural therapies and nutrition.

All medical schools had limited resources and were struggling financially. Many U.S. doctors went to Europe to gain a real foundation for medical practice and teaching.

By 1900, Rockefeller owned nearly 90% of the oil companies in the U.S. He decided he could make even more money if he developed petrochemicals into medicines, fertilizers, and pesticides. He approached allopathic medical schools with the proposition that he would build hospitals and laboratories for them if they agreed not to teach any natural therapies—even nutrition—in their medical schools.

Although Rockefeller was obsessed with extending his life by having the best diet and healthy lifestyle, he knew natural therapies were competition for his new medicines, so he wanted to do everything he could to discredit them. He insisted on having one of his people sit on the board of allopathic medical schools to ensure compliance.

In 1910, he built the Rockefeller Institute and Hospital on York Avenue and 66th Street. (This was the same Rockefeller Institute I could see from my dorm room window in medical school.) It was the first clinical research center in the United States and is a bastion of medical discovery to this day. Simon Flexner was its first director.

That same year, the Carnegie Foundation commissioned Simon Flexner's brother, Abraham Flexner, to compile a report on medical education in the U.S. Abraham visited 155 medical schools, about half of which focused on various natural therapies (including homeopathy and naturopathy), submitting his report to Congress. The study found all medical schools deficient in every respect, including laboratory facilities and hospitals. He found both administrative disorganization and a complete lack of educational standards in all medical schools.

Since its inception in 1847, the American Medical Association (AMA) represented only allopathic medical doctors and had been trying to discredit other forms of therapy, including homeopathy, without much success. However, that changed when Rockefeller entered the picture.

Thanks to the 1910 Flexner Report and Rockefeller's contributions to allopathic medical schools, Congress set accreditation standards that favored them. Almost all other medical schools were forced to close without accreditation and funding. Discrediting other medical traditions cut down on competition and demonized natural therapies to the point where people were ashamed to use them.

Rockefeller was a complex individual. Descended from a highly religious family on his mother's side, Rockefeller was a devout Christian and made significant contributions to worthwhile health-care projects, including eradicating hookworm in Alabama between 1909 and 1914.

But he also was descended from a reprobate on his father's side. Before Rockefeller was born, his father moved his pregnant mistress in with his pregnant wife and then left them both to fend for themselves while he sold snake oil and did what he wanted. J.D. Rockefeller was also a professed racist and eugenicist. Testing his petrochemicals on human subjects did not bother him at all.

Rockefeller and IG Farben

ROCKEFELLER'S DEPENDENTS CONTINUED HIS involvement in medicine beyond bribing allopathic medical schools. In 1939, they bought the controlling interest in IG Farben, Germany's largest pharmaceutical/chemical company, to test the petrochemicals.

IG Farben tested Rockefeller's petrochemicals on patients in hospitals for the chronically ill and, even after his death, on the inhabitants of concentration camps such as Auschwitz. Farben even had a pharmacist stationed at Auschwitz for this very task. These drugs inflicted great suffering on the people taking them.

In the U.S., Rockefeller went further to establish his hold on medi-cal treatment. Along with the American Medical Association (AMA), the American Cancer Society, the American Heart Association, and others, he took aggressive measures to prevent natural therapies from being taught or used in this country, largely because these natural therapies—which included diet or nutritional therapy, meditation, and exercise—were cheap and made little or no money.

Though allopathic doctors have long sought to discredit natural therapies to promote their own brand, allopathic medicine's war on natural therapies introduced a malignant and dangerous practice. The result is that most patients today don't even know there is a choice.

Even worse, most doctors are not aware of how they facilitate fraud. They debate the ethics of not telling patients the absolute truth about everything so they won't get sued, but they do not see the shocking immorality in failing to be truthful about the range of treatment possibilities available to patients with different conditions, including incorporating natural therapies like an anti-inflammatory diet and regular exercise and stretching in their treatment planning at all levels.

Most doctors I have known through the years were really good guys who were so indoctrinated into the modern medical ethos that they did not recognize what they were doing. Few know how J.D. Rockefeller changed the course of medicine in this country, and not always for the good.

But that was before American medicine became primarily a business, and doctors employed by the business were expected to make money by ordering more tests and spending less time talking to patients.

"*The art of healing comes from nature, not from the physician. Therefore, the physician must start from nature, with an open mind.*"
— PARACELSUS

"*Natural forces within us are the true healers of disease.*"
— HIPPOCRATES

CHAPTER EIGHTEEN

How Money Dominates AMA Resistance to Natural Therapies

The AMA continues its questionable practices up to the present day. Beginning in 1933, JAMA published tobacco advertisements, stating that it had done so only "after careful consideration of the extent to which cigarettes were used by physicians in practice."

The tobacco industry became the AMA's largest advertiser, and its implicit endorsement of tobacco products allowed companies like Camel to proclaim slogans such as, "More doctors smoke Camels than any other cigarette."

Of course, during this period of heavy tobacco and industry influence, the AMA defeated the health care reform proposals of both President Franklin Roosevelt and Harry Truman using the specter of "creeping socialism" that would bring "debased standards of medical care." What they really feared was making less money for doctors and themselves.

The Pharmaceutical Research and Manufacturers of America (PhRMA), a lobbying group established in 1958, spent millions opposing many aspects of health reform. Universal healthcare insurance plans might pay less for proprietary drugs or only pay for cheaper generic drugs.

At least a fifth of the AMA's budget was derived from drug companies. In addition to unsubstantiated ads in its publications, the AMA sold information about doctors themselves, spanning everything from detailed biographic information to a doctor's prescription-writing history. The drug companies used this information to market their products to doctors aggressively. Controversial drugs posing significant risks to patients were marketed to doctors using information given to them by the AMA.

Throughout the 21st century, the AMA continued to sell information to pharmaceutical companies, which used that information to promote unsafe drugs to doctors. In 2001, the *New York Times* reported that the AMA generated $20 million a year from these sales to drug companies. In 2006, that number climbed to $40 million; in 2007, it was reported to be $45 million.[41]

So, while the AMA claims to represent medicine and doctors, it's also tethered to the drug industry, medical insurance, medical device, and hospital industry, and making money. There is no evidence that they are out to improve healthcare for the nation or address optimal healing for anyone.

The AMA and other health organizations continue to donate millions of dollars to political campaigns to impede natural therapies. The AMA, the American Cancer Society, the American Heart Association, and even the NIH and the FDA have all been trashing or trying to discredit natural therapies for years.

Lest we should ask, "If what you eat can cure cancer, why take

---

41   Sidney M. Wolfe, M.D., Editor, Health Letter, "The American Medical Association and Its Dubious Revenue Streams," 2012: Vol. 28, No. 11.

all those drugs that can give you another cancer in years to come and make you sick in the meantime?"

Instead, these organizations are propped up by big money, often supported by unethical or ignorant doctors who have profited from the overdiagnosis and overmedication of an unwitting public.

In 1986, the AMA targeted chiropractors. Even though spinal manipulation has been used in many cultures for thousands of years, the AMA portrayed chiropractors as cults and tried to prevent doctors from referring patients to them.

They were unsuccessful, and in 1986, the courts found the AMA guilty of conspiring against chiropractic practitioners. Still, these efforts continue today.

Today, the AMA is the third-largest lobbying group in Washington, mainly supporting the private insurance industry. This may explain why the AMA has opposed universal health insurance, even though presidents of both parties have recommended it for over a hundred years.

Numerous books have documented the AMA's unscrupulous nature, but its efforts persist. Even EBM (evidence-based medicine) may be an attempt to use science to discredit natural therapies such as those practiced by orthomolecular psychiatry and functional medicine, which seek to treat the cause of disease rather than just control symptoms.

Because the medical establishment cannot find a way to evaluate these treatment modalities in an official double-blind trial, it misses the benefits of various forms of holistic medicine.

By saying that a treatment is only valid if it has been subjected to a double-blind study, more complex advances that cannot be boiled down to one factor are automatically dismissed. And those treatments that don't make money for anyone don't inspire spending the money to study them.

For many years, cancer specialists and others have resisted natural therapies like diet. The rationale for this criticism has been: "If standard cancer treatment is delayed, the patient may die." But that rationale fails to consider the many benefits of natural therapies, their capacity to aid healing, and their anti-cancer properties.

In 2010, I ran across a book that discussed the numerous natural therapies the American medical profession has blocked or discredited over the years. In that book, I read about Dr. Max Gerson.

Max Gerson Denied Ability to Practice in the U.S.

ONE OF THE 20TH-CENTURY doctors who used diet and other natural therapies to treat cancer was Dr. Max Gerson. He used food to effect a cure. Dr. Albert Schweitzer came from Africa to Germany to be treated for cancer by Dr. Gerson. When Hitler began persecuting Jews, Dr. Gerson, who was Jewish, left Germany and came to this country, but Gerson was not allowed to practice in the U.S. because the medical establishment had outlawed using any treatment other than chemotherapy to treat cancer in this country.

Since he did not use the standard American chemotherapy, Dr. Gerson had to move his practice to Mexico to treat patients. To this day, his natural therapies are used to treat cancer patients, but still in Mexico.

In this country, Gerson's treatments were discredited, as were other natural anti-cancer substances like marijuana.[42] The excuse has always been that using natural therapy delays the start of real

---

42 Archaeological evidence suggests that plant-based medicines date back to the Paleolithic age. However, in terms of recorded medicines, Cannabis sativa is one of the oldest, having been discovered in 2700 BCE.

cancer treatment (chemotherapy.) Rather than embrace the range of available therapies and study what works best for which patients, the medical profession just took a hard line on all treatments involving natural therapy, even food.

As far as I can tell, Dr. Gerson's treatments helped patients feel better and live more comfortable lives for a longer period than traditional chemotherapy. But, of course, cancer treatment in the U.S. has always been about curing the disease and killing the cancer cells, not about making patients better able to fight off cancer on their own or be healthier and more comfortable in their last days.

Patients tend to feel the doctor has given up on them when chemotherapy no longer works. Too often, when chemotherapy is no longer effective, cancer patients are offered toxic experimental treatments to kill their cancer cells, not therapy to make their last days healthier and more comfortable.

Fortunately, today, there are more offerings in the cancer arena than were accepted in the 20th century. Many professionals advocate an anti-cancer diet to prevent recurrence, and hospice is making patients' lives easier in the end.

Five states have even found a way to allow patients to determine when they have suffered enough. Still, we live in a country that is obsessed with youth and wants to deny that aging and death are in the picture for us all.

Still, I did not understand how effective natural therapies could be forbidden in this country until I read about John D. Rockefeller and what his embrace of allopathic medicine did to medical treatment in America and read about the AMA's assault on natural therapies.

I did not understand why modern health insurance would only cover concrete treatments like tests, surgery, and medications until I learned about Rockefeller's part of the puzzle.

Insurance in this country is an important part of the healthcare takeover by pharmaceutical companies and allopathic medicine. In Germany, both natural therapies and Western medical interventions are paid for. Even today, homeopathy is covered by the government in Germany and Britain. But in America, natural therapies—even psychotherapy—are often not covered by insurance.

Even so, many have slipped back into acceptability in the U.S. under the label of alternative, complementary, or integrative medicine (CAM). In fact, in the 21st century, CAM has grown into a multibillion-dollar industry in the U.S. Still, as a nation, we are at the mercy of a medical system that has co-opted science to support its own existence and to discredit any competition.

The American medical system is not set up to ferret out the best and safest treatments for each condition. After all, who will pay for double-blind studies of natural therapies, especially when the standard for discounting the effectiveness of any treatment is the placebo effect? Who is going to study the negative aspects of a drug and compare those toxic or even lethal aspects to a natural therapy for the same condition with the same vigor they used to study the hoped-for positive effects? And who will promote natural therapies with the same vigor as all that TV ad money?

Drug companies control the market, pay for studies of their drugs, and support many prominent doctors who have benefited from their largesse and thus perpetuate the system. Organized medicine in this country has been fighting natural therapies for more than two hundred years, and the pattern is so entrenched it seems reasonable.

Modern medicine has accomplished some amazing advances, but at what cost to a suffering public? Even the food we eat is now based on petrochemicals, not on products of the sun. As a people, we are embedded in a culture in which money and big business dominate every industry, including food, medicine, and politics. Doctors have become like the fish who do not know they're wet because he has become one with the water.

But attitudes are beginning to shift in some places. The word about natural therapies is getting out, leading to change. Open-heart surgery and the placement of stents to reduce the likelihood of a heart attack are now being joined by lifestyle changes in diet and exercise, in addition to medication.

We now know that daily exercise and a plant-based, natural diet without processed foods can actually reverse heart disease in a fairly short time, even if long-standing damage does not completely disappear. We also know the right diet can prevent, if not reverse, most cancers that have an environmental cause. And we have learned that a plant-based diet without processed foods can affect the immune system and the type of bacteria that grow in the gut.

Even the Mayo and Cleveland Clinics offer some alternative and complementary therapies to their patients because they seem to be safe and appear to work. According to the Cleveland Clinic website, available integrative therapies include Acupuncture, Brain Health, Chinese Herbal Therapy, Chiropractic Therapy, Culinary Medicine, Disease Reversal Programs, Holistic Psychotherapy, Hypnotherapy, Integrative Medicine Consults—a holistic approach to managing chronic symptoms, Interactive Guided Imagery; Lifestyle U—a weight and lifestyle management program, Lifestyle Medicine Consults—medical consultation to manage chronic symptoms through lifestyle changes, Living Well—after breast cancer or prostate cancer, Massotherapy—massage therapy; Mind/Body Coaching—relaxation practice, Nutrition Consults, Recovery Programs—for those suffering from alcohol and substance abuse, Reiki, Shared Medical Appointments—unique appointments held in the company of others who share similar health concerns, and Yoga. These are the practices, techniques, and services patients find most helpful and are willing to pay for.

Homeopathy Today

AFTER ROCKEFELLER AND THE AMA targeted natural therapies, people in the United States were embarrassed to use them for many years. However, they eventually made a comeback. Today, homeopathy, in particular, is still going strong despite the continued furor against its use.

Very popular in Great Britain and a special favorite of the royal family, homeopathy is now a multibillion-dollar enterprise. The British National Health program even uses about 1% of its budget to support homeopathy.

In Germany, homeopathy has always been covered by the government and insurance, along with standard medical treatment. Homeopathy use continues to grow worldwide. In 2007, Great Britain spent 62 million dollars on homeopathy treatments, Germany spent 346 million, and France spent 408 million. However, that year, the United States topped them all by spending 2.9 billion on homeopathy.[43]

Though criticized by many, the growing popularity of homeopathy and other alternative therapies seems undeniable. Many well-researched books dismiss alternative therapies because they only encourage a placebo effect, without realizing they are dismissing the ultimate benefit of all treatment—that it allows the body to heal itself, so patients can get on with their lives.

Today, doctors and others still want to separate "real" medicine

---

43   Key technical issues of quality impacting the safety of Homeopathic medicines: apps.who.int/gb/ebwha/pdf_files/A62/A62_R13-en.pdf.

from healing based on what we now call the "placebo effect." However, this is a false choice, as we will see. Next, we will get to what brings about healing and the much-misunderstood placebo effect.

"There can be no transforming of darkness into light and of apathy into movement without emotion."
— CARL GUSTAV JUNG

"Memory is always faulty. Emotions are always true."
— UNKNOWN

"Yet this placebo effect, a belief in the cure, is the crux of the healing role physicians play in the progression of illness to healing. Doctors have been so convinced that any improvement attributable to the placebo effect is just trickery that they tend to discount the lessons of the placebo effect throughout history."
— SUMTER CARMICHAEL

The Power of the Mind to Influence the Body: Emotions and Healing; Enter the Placebo Effect

I was introduced to the placebo effect early in my medical career. As a medical student, part of my job was to examine patients, draw blood, and run medical tests such as EKGs on the heart.

One day, I was finishing an EKG on one of the patients when she sat up and began thanking me. "I feel so much better, Doctor," she said. "Thank you!"

The patient was an unsophisticated woman who did not know I was just a student running a test, but she did look vastly relieved. Clearly, she did feel better. Was she just less anxious because the test was over? I had no idea, but the patient definitely thought I was administering a treatment, and it had worked.

As a student intent on pursuing psychiatry, I was especially interested in the dynamics of the doctor-patient relationship and how often doctors and patients alike misinterpret what transpires in any given interaction.

Too often, doctors tend to think confused and delirious patients are just being difficult. Sobbing patients are just hysterical or have personality disorders. And the patient who felt better after her EKG was considered just a "stupid" female. But I saw these various patient responses as clues to be explored, just like any other symptom.

The EKG machine, with its many cords and attachments, which I carefully connected to the patient's body, was bound to impress and inspire someone new to the medical game. It provided reassurance, along with my touch, that made the patient feel better. This experience was only the beginning of my journey to see how some physicians could make patients feel better while others tended to worsen the situation.

It took me many years to fully understand the placebo effect. However, I have never been able to understand why so many physicians resist the idea that it is so beneficial.

How Healing Works

MOST CONDITIONS, INCLUDING MANY infections and injuries, heal by themselves and don't require doctor intervention. In fact, only 20% of problems doctors treat actually need modern medicine's intervention. And that's part of the difficulty. The other 80% of problems that patients bring to doctors require little intervention other than reassurance and encouragement to get back to doing what works.

Increased weakness on one visit to my neurologist is a good example. My legs were weaker because I had not been exercising as much, because I'd been sick all spring with one infection after another. All my doctor could think of when I was weaker was that my MS had become active or my spinal cord was being pinched. So, I needed an MRI to help him decide whether to give me a pill for the MS or have surgery for the pinched nerve. I declined.

I knew 80% of pain problems are musculoskeletal in origin. Even pain problems that re-emerge periodically, such as my husband's back pain after sitting too long writing his book, fall into the 80%.

In such cases, all doctors can really do is perform an unnecessary procedure or order tests to be sure the problem is not something else that actually does require intervention. Were they to investigate what the patient was doing and how much exercise and stretching they had been doing, they might have been able to go in a different direction.

Doctors get frustrated when patients appear with conditions the body will cure on its own, or, even worse, when patients complain of physical symptoms that result from stress, anxiety, or depression, all of which can lead to changes in behavior that affect health.

In general, doctors tend to regard emotion as an inconvenience or an impediment to their real task of seeking out real diseases and providing real treatments. This view results from doctors' overly simplistic approach to the body and health. Also, seeing the body as a machine is an unconscious way of dealing with anxiety, which may be a factor as well.

Doctors and researchers have discounted for many years how emotions and beliefs affect behavior and health. Even though the healing effects of heartening beliefs and helpful, positive emotions have been recognized for thousands of years, modern doctors have tended to see optimism and the placebo effect as unnecessary in caring for patients.

Rather than recognize that these things are at the heart of all healing, doctors have tended to believe that when they give a medicine or other treatment to a patient, this real treatment affects real change, not the patient's frame of mind or behavior. Doctors tend to regard the placebo effect as merely giving the patient a sugar pill to trick them or placate them. However, the placebo phenomenon has nothing to do with trickery and has much to do with the real miracle of healing: positive emotions and proactive behaviors.

Understanding How Emotions Affect Healing

EMOTIONS ARE NOT JUST how we feel. Emotions also lead to certain behaviors. For example, depression does not just mean you feel sad. Depression causes you to withdraw from friends and your usual interests and activities and to focus on how bad you feel, perhaps even ruminating about suicide.

Depression means you lose interest in sex, in sports, in people. You care less about all the things that were once important to you. At the same time, you don't take as much care of yourself. You may eat too much of the worst foods or stop eating altogether. You may stay home in bed rather than exercising and getting together with friends.

All emotions, including depression, lead to chemical changes in the body. Negative emotions tend to make you feel worse and less likely to make an effort, while positive emotions tend to make you feel better and, therefore, do better. Feeling good can lead to behaviors that encourage healing.

So, when we see a placebo affecting a change in emotion, far from being trivial, this placebo is making a significant change in our brain and body chemistry and behavior. Beneficial chemistry and healthy behavior are what help us get well. If you're sick and don't take care of yourself, you may get worse.

Believing in your doctor and your treatment will make you more optimistic and more likely to take better care of yourself by getting up and getting back to healthy living. Remember, healing comes from healthy behavior. You have to act well to get well.

So, What's the Difficulty?

THE PROBLEM IS THAT the dictionary defines "placebo" as: a harmless pill, medicine, or procedure prescribed more for the psychological benefit to the patient than for any physiological effect, a substance that has no therapeutic effect, used as a control in testing new drugs, or a measure designed merely to calm or please someone. Intertwined in this kind of definition is the suggestion of trickery.

The word "placebo" was coined in the 18th century and is derived from the Latin "placeō," meaning "to please." As I said in my 2013 book, *Heal*: "Placebos have nothing to do with deception or lying. They have to do with finding a story, or an activity that the patient can relate to that helps him or her live with the reality of what is happening."

Humans are symbolic beings. They live with symbolic constructs that help them master particular tasks. When we are sick, we go to the doctor who gives us a pill to make us well. The pill may have no effect on our particular problem, but our belief in the healing effect of that pill starts the healing process.

The question is not about truth or reality; it is about survival and finding constructs that facilitate healing that do not lead to depression or a sense of hopelessness and despair, which can make us worse. Today, we have the science to back this up.

Remember, the body is programmed to survive. Too often, we forget that the body is programmed to heal on its own. Even when the surgeon cuts, the body heals the wound. Most illnesses, pains, bleeding, and vomiting heal on their own. Only a limited number of conditions cannot heal by themselves, or will likely result in death or permanent disability if no medical intervention takes place.

Reasons for the Confusion Over the Placebo Effect

PART OF THE CONFUSION over the placebo effect lies with how science has handled emotions. René Descartes (1596-1650) approached the body like a machine. He relegated emotions to the province of the supernatural or religion, which meant the medical profession could dismiss them. Emotions were not concrete enough to be studied like the physical body. Yet emotions have a stunning effect on the body, our behavior, and our chemical makeup.

The second reason for this confusion about the placebo effect is how "sham pills," or "placebos," were introduced into medicine. The term "placebo effect" entered the medical lexicon after World War II when the anesthesiologist Henry K. Beecher discovered he could use shots of sugar water when he ran out of opium, and soldiers still got pain relief.

While belief may have played a role in pain relief, the experience of injecting opium via a syringe also set the stage for a "conditioned response." Beecher urged the use of this "sham pill," or "placebo," in double-blind tests on new and old medications to assess their real, not imagined effects.

The Misunderstood Sugar Pill

One reason many doctors have long been skeptical about the benefit of the placebo effect in their treatments is that they thought patients could be "fooled" into feeling better by sugar pills or shots. They failed to recognize the difference between a conditioned response and the beneficial effect of believing in one's treatment, the placebo effect. Replacing opiates with sugar water produced a conditioned response, much like with Pavlov's dogs. The placebo effect in recovery from illness is a different issue.

In 1889, Ivan Pavlov, a Russian physiologist, demonstrated that by ringing a bell each time food is put in front of a dog, the dog can be made to salivate just by ringing the bell without any food. This is called a "conditioned reflex" or "classical conditioning."

Similarly, if you give a patient a shot of morphine for pain and then replace the morphine with sugar water, the patient will associate the shot with pain relief and respond accordingly. This is a conditioned response from getting the shot, not a placebo effect.

Too often, a placebo is defined as receiving a benefit from something with no obvious medical potency, like giving a sham pill in a placebo-controlled trial.[44] However, placebo effects do not result from associated behavior; they result from a belief in the treatment. Placebo effects result from the healing effects of the doctor-patient relationship, the so-called art of medicine.

The Opiate Response

ANOTHER MISUNDERSTANDING THAT HAS contributed to the confusion about pain and the placebo effect is that many doctors, as well as patients, don't know that opiates only treat the emotional aspects of pain. Opiates do not affect the pain threshold. Opiates do not make you hurt less. The discomfort is still present after taking an opiate; the patient just does not care because they are no longer suffering and unable to focus on anything else.

Dr. Beecher also demonstrated how meaning and emotion determine the amount of pain one has, as well as the effect of opiates. During WWII, Beecher observed that conscious soldiers who were

44   A placebo-controlled trial is a study in which one group gets the active treatment (the test substance), while the other group gets an inert substance or placebo. Everything else is kept the same in the two groups so no one conducting the study knows which group is which. That way, any difference in the outcome can be attributed to the active treatment.

wounded and being evacuated from the beach had very little pain and did not require opiates. In contrast, soldiers with minor wounds who were being patched up and sent back into battle had a lot of pain and required a lot of opiates.

The Placebo Effect and Money

THE FINAL REASON FOR confusion about the benefit of the placebo effect is that we live in a world dominated by money. Natural therapies using the placebo effect tend to be less expensive and readily available. Meanwhile, pharmaceutical companies spend a lot of money promoting their drugs, and physicians are trained to prescribe drugs rather than natural therapies or even dietary changes.

If doctors get paid by ordering tests rather than talking to patients, then that is what they'll do. If they get paid by writing a prescription for pills rather than spending time sorting out what exercise or food may be contributing to the problem, then that is what they tend to do as well.

A Visit to China Expanded My Understanding of Belief

IN 1982, I WENT to China as a guest of the Chinese government to see how Chinese physicians treat depression. At the time, I saw China as an alien world, far more different from the United States and our ways than any other place I had encountered.

While in China, I observed a patient having a lung removed under acupuncture anesthesia. At the end of the surgery, the patient got up from the operating table and walked into the next room.

I asked the Chinese surgeon showing us around, "Do you generally use acupuncture or Western anesthesia during surgery?"

"Oh, Western anesthesia!" he replied. "You can't take a scared patient into the operating room and just stick acupuncture needles in him. It takes a carefully prepared patient to respond to acupuncture. He must believe he won't feel pain!"

Eureka! A light bulb went off in my head.

The phrase "Christianity is only for Christians" has always bothered me. What kind of God would discriminate against people who had never heard of Him? Suddenly, listening to this Chinese surgeon, I realized God doesn't discriminate against anyone. God provides lots of ways to get relief from pain. But Christianity is only for Christians because it only works for those who believe in it! Like the placebo effect or acupuncture, you respond to the doctor's treatment if you believe it will work.

Modern Science Rolls Back the Curtain on the Placebo Effect

MODERN SCIENCE HAS DEMONSTRATED how placebos work. The placebo effect changes the immune system and other systems in the body related to healing. If we believe in our treatment, we are more apt to activate our immune system and other healthy mechanisms that facilitate our recovery, including participating in health-promoting behavior.

As Norman Cousins observed forty years ago, belief and a positive attitude facilitate healing mechanisms in the body. Although he did not use the term, he was talking about the placebo effect. Fear and depression tend to suppress the healing effects. Interventions producing negative expectations and results are now called "nocebos."

Critics of alternative therapies (so-called placebo therapies) say alternative practitioners are not being honest when they do not tell patients about the worst possible outcomes. These critics don't realize that informing patients of the worst possible outcomes may protect the doctor from getting sued, but it may not benefit the patient. If the expected outcome is so negative, perhaps the doctor should not be performing the procedure in the first place.

But even bad news can be presented positively. When praying, one does not announce, "Now, most people think this is worthless, but it can't hurt!" When the doctor fails to recognize the power of belief in his treatments and only thinks in terms of what a surgery, shot, or pill will do, he limits his ability to heal the patient and ensure his recovery.

Hospice

ONE EXAMPLE OF THE body's ability to benefit from a positive approach is hospice. Medical care tends to focus only on attacking the disease. If the patient dies, the doctor has failed. Often, patients think of hospice as meaning doctors are giving up. If doctors don't have any other drugs to try to keep them alive, patients are terrified. But hospice actually focuses on making patients more comfortable so they don't suffer as much and can live more productive days before the end.

While the doctor's heroic treatments aimed at delaying the inevitable end make patients very sick, hospice offers the great benefit of a peaceful end of life, not one shortened by toxic chemicals. It also opens the door to the healing effects of the body. There are many stories of people at the end of cancer treatment who actually get better.

Science Shows the Placebo Effect Can Make Real Changes in the Body

IN THE PAST FIVE years, science has shown what changes occur in the body with the placebo effect and who is most likely to respond. We have known for some time that about 30% of people are "placebo responders." With positive suggestions, this percentage can be increased to about 60 percent.

Brain studies in the past few years have demonstrated differences in the brain structures of placebo responders.[45] These neural traits were present before exposure to the placebo treatment, and most remained stable during and after treatment.

Furthermore, psychological traits such as interior awareness and openness also predicted the magnitude of response to a placebo. These results shed light on psychological, neuroanatomical, and neurophysiological principles determining placebo responses in chronic pain patients. This suggests the long-term beneficial effects of a placebo are partially predictable.[46]

Other brain studies have demonstrated that certain personality traits are more common among placebo responders. In particular, placebo responders have been found to have more optimism, suggestibility, empathy, and neuroticism (anxiousness). In contrast, nocebo effects have been linked to personality traits such as pessimism, anxiety, and thinking that everything is a catastrophe.

In addition, expectations play a major role in the effectiveness of a placebo. If you expect to do better, you are more likely to do so than if you don't expect to do well. This may support the observation that what people believe about their health has more of an effect on how well they do than the actual results of objective tests.

Recent studies have also shown that placebos release endorphins,

---

45   Subcortical limbic volume asymmetry, sensorimotor cortical thickness, and functional coupling of the prefrontal regions, anterior cingulate, and peri-aqueductal gray were all predictive of a response to a placebo.

46   Etienne Vachon-Presseau, Sara E. Berger, Taha B. Abdullah, Lejian Huang, Guillermo A. Cecchi, James W. Griffith, Thomas J. Schnitzer, "A. Vania Apkarian Nature Communications," Volume 9, 2018: article 3397. REF Brain and psychological determinants of placebo pill response in chronic pain patients.

the hormones in our nervous system that address pain, stress, depression, and anxiety. Endorphins are naturally occurring opiates. Placebos also bring about changes in the dopamine system.

Dopamine is a neurotransmitter in the brain associated with pleasure and good feelings. Since Parkinson's disease and asthma both involve a deficit of dopamine, this explains why placebos can even help manage the symptoms of these conditions as well.

Since placebos produce real changes in the brain, and affirmative suggestions encourage these changes further, we can now understand how positive expectations enhance the healing process while negative expectations do the opposite.

The important point here is that the placebo effect has both biological and psychological roots. It's time to stop seeing the placebo effect as merely a control in a placebo-controlled drug trial to separate the real effect of a medicine or intervention from a fake one.

Either way, the question we need to focus on as physicians and as a society increasingly charged with responsibility for its own healing is what best facilitates the body's efforts to get well—be it surgery, medicine, food, exercise, meditation, massage, hypnosis, psychotherapy, prayer, the doctor-patient relationship or other natural therapies.

This also means assessing not only the beneficial effects of treatment modalities, especially drugs, compared to a placebo, but also the toxic and even lethal effects of standard medical treatments compared to natural therapies. (Have you seen all those TV ads?)

The Impact of What the Doctor Tells the Patient

DOCTORS DEBATE THE ETHICS of lying to patients about the nature of the drugs and other treatments they receive. They are also wary of getting sued and want to structure communication to protect themselves. And recently, doctors have discovered that placebos work even if patients know they are taking a placebo.

In other words, a double-blind study does not have to be conducted to assess the placebo effect. Doctors speculate that something about the interaction with the doctor facilitates the healing process. Eureka!

In the past, doctors told patients what they thought they should hear, even sometimes failing to tell them they had cancer. This approach suggests they knew their patients would do better if they expected a positive outcome. This has changed in modern times thanks to malpractice suits against doctors. Still, presenting any information to patients must be given in the most constructive way to not damage the patient's ability to heal.

Unconscious Defenses Limit Doctors, Too

DOCTORS ARE HUMAN BEINGS, and like René Descartes, they have relied on concrete thinking (their unconscious defense mechanisms) to deal with their anxieties. That's why, even with scientific evidence about placebos, it is hard for doctors to give up trying to separate real treatments for illness from the effect of the body's curative mechanism and the power of the doctor-patient relationship to further healing.

One reason for that is the view of psychologists that our conscious mind overrides the unconscious mind. In other words, if we consciously learned something like how to drive a car, that could become unconscious, as it does. They did not countenance that we are born with an unconscious mind that keeps us alive and safe, for the most part.

Acknowledging the unconscious mind would threaten the notion that we as human beings have free will and are making conscious choices to do good or do ill. So they have denied evidence of the unconscious or attributed that wisdom to a higher being, such as God. That's displacement, another unconscious defense mechanism against anxiety.

How About a Placebo Pill?

SOME DOCTORS HAVE EVEN theorized that once we know what chemicals are involved in the placebo effect, pharmaceutical companies can make a placebo pill. But we already have such a pill in opiates. Our problem is that we, Americans, have become too dependent on taking pills for pain and other discomforts to the exclusion of other activities.

As of 2012, Americans were consuming 80% of the world's pain medicines (opiates). In fact, we have become too dependent on pills, shots, and surgery for everything instead of using the God-given gifts that help us stay healthy and recover from illness.

It's fine to say we should expand the placebo part of drug trials, but what about comparing an alternative or natural therapy to the new medication, looking at the side effects and toxic effects of both? Without including what we know to be beneficial, we are not offering the best to our patients.

The Magic of Healing

WHEN I CUT MYSELF, I keep the wound clean by washing it and putting on clean dressings, but it is the body that heals the cut. When I get a cold, I take Nyquil, zinc, and Airborne to shorten the duration of my illness, but the body's defense mechanisms fighting off the germs cause me to get well. When a surgeon operates and closes the incision with stitches or glue, the body mends the cut.

Suppose I was told to drink a glass of water every day at six a.m.

to heal what ails me. If I did so faithfully, I might also do all the other things to care for myself that would allow the body to heal itself. If I ignored the effect of water and continued going out drinking alcohol with my buddies, staying up late, eating junk food, and not getting enough rest, I might get worse. This placebo effect facilitates healing through the conscious and unconscious things we do as we recover.

Doctors Wrestle With the Placebo Effect

WHEN I WAS ON the Multiple Sclerosis Society Advisory Board in my forties, someone wrote an article about the benefits of exercise for patients with multiple sclerosis for the MS Society's magazine. The physicians on the advisory board were very negative about the article.

"That's all the placebo effect," one said.

I spoke up, "You know, the history of medical treatment is the history of the placebo effect. Everything has a placebo effect."

"Yes, even the new medicine for MS, Interferon, has a placebo effect!" Dr. Barth, the multiple sclerosis specialist on the committee, chimed in.

"It does?" the other physicians gasped.

They thought they had finally found a real treatment for multiple sclerosis with interferon. Dr. Barth assured them, "Oh, yes, Interferon has a placebo effect." All the physicians were astonished.

"When Harry Potter asks Dumbledore if what he's experiencing is real or just in his head, Dumbledore responds: 'Of course it is happening inside your head, Harry, but why on earth should that mean it is not real?'"
— HARRY POTTER AND THE DEATHLY HALLOWS - J.K. ROWLING

"People think that epilepsy is divine simply because they don't have any idea what causes epilepsy. But I believe that someday we will understand what causes epilepsy, and at that moment, we will cease to believe that it's divine. And so it is with everything in the universe"
— HIPPOCRATES

CHAPTER TWENTY

The Truth About Healing and Spirituality

From the beginning of time, humans have attributed events they did not understand to the gods. This is especially true in medicine and the mysterious realm of sickness and health, life and death.

Religious institutions have always associated themselves with life-and-death issues: birth, sickness, and dying. Furthermore, from time to time throughout history, even into modern times, certain individuals have had a remarkable ability to bring about healing in others.

Greek healer-priests who established themselves as medical practitioners were first mentioned in recorded history in the West in 1500 BCE. They believed life energy and the spirit were one with the divine. These gifted healers inspired people to believe their abilities came from heaven.

In 1000 BCE, the Egyptian healer Imhotep was so famous for his healing ways that he was deified as the Egyptian God of Healing after his death. The sick could pray to him and be healed.

Jesus of Nazareth was another gifted healer, perhaps the greatest natural healer of all time. He cured both physical and spiritual illnesses: blindness, lameness, deafness, insanity, and leprosy. His ability to heal people was so great that, like other healers before him, his power was attributed to God. After his death, his disciples were able to heal in his name, demonstrating the power of belief, if not of God.

This healing in the name of Jesus continued into the Middle Ages. The Roman Catholic Church used the belief in God to manipulate the people, even selling saints' relics to relieve pain.[47] The church made money by selling bones and other relics of the saints, purported to relieve pain.[48]

Seeking Practical Interventions to Cure Disease

SOME HEALERS IN ANCIENT times also sought practical ideas to explain illness and treatment. Hippocrates (460-375 BCE) is regarded by many as the father of medicine. He considered himself a pragmatist and introduced the idea of the four humors (blood, phlegm, black bile, and yellow bile) as the cause of disease. He was also considered a great natural healer.

Galen (129-216 AD) was the most famous doctor of his time, perhaps because he was a master at self-promotion. A Greek trained in Alexandria, Egypt, Galen moved to Rome, where he became a prolific writer. Galen was a firm devotee of Asclepius, the god of

47   The Roman Catholic Church took advantage of people's belief to bring them into the Church as the only way to heaven. They forbade birth control to grow their membership and retained their wealth by making their priests stay unmarried and poor. Monks and priests continued to have sex and father children but had no responsibility for those children. Townspeople hired prostitutes to send to the monasteries to protect their young girls and boys.

48   It seems that the urge to make money drives human behavior, whether in religious institutions, politics, business, or the medical profession. There are always dedicated priests, leaders, and healers, but money tends to bring deceit and corruption into every area of human endeavor.

healing, and his office was in a temple devoted to Asclepius. Like Hippocrates, he espoused the theory of the four humors as the cause of disease, but he also believed illness was caused and could be cured by the gods.

Galen's writings promoting the humoral theory of disease and their treatments were popular well past the Middle Ages. Treatment of the four humors to restore balance consisted of bleeding, enemas, and emetics to cause vomiting. Well into the late 19th century, doctors were still unknowingly killing their patients with bloodletting and toxic substances.

Science Begins to Question the Church

THE RENAISSANCE ENCOURAGED CURIOSITY, investigation, and discovery, leading to the modern scientific approach. People began questioning old beliefs and using experiments and mathematics to understand the natural world. As a result, new discoveries were made, and some old beliefs were proven wrong.

Following the Renaissance, a belief in scientific healing began to take precedence over a belief in spiritual healing. As faith in spiritual healing waned, so too did its effectiveness. As faith in scientific healing grew, so too did the scientific power to heal. Rationalism and a focus on the tangible became the basis for medicine.

Descartes Treated the Body Like a Machine

ALTHOUGH EARLIER PHYSICIANS AND philosophers identified both concrete and spiritual elements responsible for illness and healing, we credit the start of scientific thinking about the body to the mathematician and scientist René Descartes (1596-1650). Descartes declared that the body was like a machine and could be studied and treated as such.

Descartes assigned emotional and spiritual issues to the province of the supernatural or the divine. Emotions were regarded as weaknesses of the mentally feeble and female members of the species. This idea not only did a great disservice to women and the poor, but it also caused physicians to overlook the important role emotions play in the healing process and, otherwise, in our lives.

Today, of course, we know that emotional and spiritual matters can profoundly affect the body and brain. Strong emotions can affect changes in the body's chemistry, as well as trigger mental and physical paralysis. Furthermore, once the emotional part of our brain is destroyed, we lose the capacity to make any decisions. Descartes is quoted as saying, "I think, therefore I am." He should have said, "I feel, therefore I am."

Descartes's flight into concrete thinking, or rationalism, has been shown to be an unconscious defense mechanism against anxiety. In her book, *The Flight to Objectivity*, Susan Bordo demonstrates how Descartes used an unconscious defense mechanism against anxiety when he latched onto treating the body as a machine.

Humankind has benefited from extricating the control of medicine from religious oversight, but since medicine still does not fully embrace the reality of healing's connection to emotion and belief, there is yet more work to be done. We will run behind until we accept how much human beings are run by unconscious mechanisms.

Indeed, this misconception has affected physician practices throughout history. Medical professionals use unconscious defenses against anxiety in their decision-making, especially when faced with life-and-death issues. Over and over again, we see unconscious defenses lead doctors to focus on concrete issues rather than contend with the uncertainty of emotions—even the uncertainty of the placebo effect.

A perfect example of this is the path psychiatry took in the 20th century into brain research rather than delving further into psycho-social issues. Seeking medications for every human condition rather than exploring unconscious dynamics, they grounded psychiatrists in concrete issues: a pill for every human condition.

I remember hearing the anxiety in the voices and proposals of my fellow psychiatrists in the 1980s when the government began cutting back on payments for psychotherapy and psychiatrists, while psychologists were pushing to be allowed to prescribe medications.

A Natural Healer Discounted by Science

In 1780, Anton Mesmer, a German physician and natural healer with a background in astronomy, appeared on the scene as a great healer. He called his healing ability "Animal Magnetism" because he believed the healing came from internal magnetism. Initially, he gave patients iron particles until he realized they were unnecessary.

So many people came to see him to be healed, he held long rods so people could touch the rods or the hem of his robe and be healed. It's said his power to heal was so strong that people could just look at him or hear his voice and be healed. His method was criticized by the medical establishment of the day as not being scientific enough.

As a result, Mesmer was run out of town and died in disgrace. Clearly, the stand science takes against those things it cannot understand is not always wise. Today, his miraculous cures are attributed to "hypnosis."[49] Hypnotizability is an inborn characteristic. About 10% of the population is highly hypnotizable, which means they can be captured by words in a lecture or on TV and instantly be changed.[50]

49   American Psychological Association (APA). Hypnosis is defined as "a state of consciousness involving focused attention and reduced peripheral awareness characterized by an enhanced capacity for response to suggestion."

50   During hypnosis a region of the brain called the dorsal anterior cingulate cortex

Again and again, throughout history, so-called "miraculous cures" have been reported. These events are deemed miraculous because people don't understand what brings about the healing.

The cures that followed a visit to a spring at Lourdes, France, is just one example. From February to July 1858, a fourteen-year-old miller's daughter in Lourdes, Bernadette Soubirous, reported eighteen apparitions of "a lady" at a nearby spring. After that, visitors to the spring appeared to be miraculously cured of their illnesses.

In 1897, the skeptical Vatican asked Jean-Martin Charcot, a well-known physician of the time, to investigate these claims. He found that tumors shrank after visits to this spring and other evidence of physical cures, in addition to various spiritual ones. Nothing was found unusual about the water in the spring.

Even in standard medical or surgical treatment, the advent of a new drug for cancer that proves generally ineffective or a surgery stopped short of completion has resulted in a physical cure. We tend to want to discount the power of belief in the healing process because we don't fully understand how it works. Even though we see the evidence over and over again, some cures just don't fit our general notion of how healing takes place.

We forget about the power of the unconscious to keep us healthy and well. In other words, the unconscious is always looking for ways to encourage our immune system and other systems of the body to secure our health. Our beliefs impact all aspects of that healing apparatus.

Like all the centuries of humans that have come before us, modern humans want certainty. Humans dislike complexity and paradox. They don't like to hear that what they assume is happening might

becomes less active.

not actually be happening or that others may see or experience something very different from what they do. They don't want to hear that neither party nor both may be perceiving the truth, deluded, or experiencing a mix of the two.

Modern, scientifically oriented physicians have long sought cures that can be separated from their spiritual or psychological components. While religion may want to deny science by saying, "God did it!" Medical practitioners too often want to deny the role of the spirit or belief in healing. Luckily, modern science is beginning to shed light on how belief affects healing.

To be fair, faith healing is not consistent enough or fast enough to appeal to modern humans who want swift, predictable answers. We have seen too many movies where miraculous cures seem instantaneous rather than gradual shifts toward growing health.

Quacks, Cults, Charlatans

FOR HUNDREDS OF YEARS—AND even in modern times—natural healers have been attacked not only by the church but also by the most prominent medical practitioners. For hundreds of years, the church burned natural healers at the stake as witches, making them the scapegoat for the pandemics that ravaged Europe. The medical establishment did its part by attacking natural healers as quacks, charlatans, and cultists.

Even though modern studies in psychology and psychiatry have demonstrated the mind's role in regulating health, many in the medical establishment continue to resist the healing effects touted by many natural healers.

Natural healers such as Mary Baker Eddy, who formed the

Christian Science Church; Edgar Cayce; Joel Goldsmith; and Caroline Myss all tapped into the mind's ability to heal the body, and they have been able to help thousands of people.

"I'll take transformational change any way it comes. One way to look at meditation is as a kind of intra-psychic technology that's been developed over thousands of years by traditions that know a lot about the mind/body connection. To call what happens 'the placebo effect' is just to give a name to something we don't understand."
— Jon Kabat-Zinn

"The greatest medicine of all is teaching people how not to need it."
— Hippocrates

Embracing Alternative Therapies: Where We Are Today In the War to Discredit Natural Therapy

Even though most alternative therapies have been around for many years, they continue to be denounced because they represent a challenge to the modern system. Most alternative therapies have been criticized because they haven't been studied for safety or efficacy, or are "no better than a placebo."

But most alternative therapies, in addition to promoting healing, also address what modern medicine calls "lifestyle issues." These are behaviors essential for good health and recovery from illness. Rather than just relying on a pill or substance to treat symptoms, they address the day-to-day activities we all need to embrace to be healthy, recover from illness, and retard deterioration as we get older.

Over the years, practitioners of alternative and complementary therapies have been accused of being frauds, charlatans, and quacks in order to discredit them, even while they were offering beneficial therapy. Today, the renewed interest in complementary and alternative treatments (CAM) appears to relate to other spiritual shifts we're seeing in American culture.

While most people in the United States identify as members of a traditional organized religion, they also increasingly embrace one or more so-called New Age beliefs, such as reincarnation, astrology, psychics, or the presence of spiritual energy in physical objects like mountains or trees.

Roughly 60% of adults in America accept at least one of these beliefs. Specifically, 40% believe in psychics and the idea that spiritual energy can be found in physical objects, while a smaller percentage express belief in reincarnation (33%) and astrology (29%).[51] These beliefs appear to correlate strongly with an interest in CAM.[52]

This only adds to the confusion and complication when evaluating the best treatment for any individual. However, it also reminds us that the scientific community may not yet fully understand many of the effects we observe in the world and the healing process.

Unfortunately, this New Age group has also aligned itself with the anti-vaccine movement. Vaccines are one of the true miracles brought about by modern medicine. They have saved humankind from illnesses that spread easily and cause widespread sickness and death. Vaccines may produce allergic reactions and other side effects, which make some wary of their use, but they have saved millions of lives.

When I was thirty-eight, I lost vision in my left eye thirty minutes after I received a flu vaccine. That particular vaccine precipitated a lot of neurological effects in those who took the shot. My symptoms

---

51   Claire Gecewicz, Facttank, Pew Research Center, 2018. "New Age Beliefs" are common among religious and nonreligious Americans.

52   Complementary and alternative medicine.

disappeared after a few days, but I did not get another flu vaccine for thirty years. Others who had a bad experience with the flu shot have also avoided them.

Still, vaccines are lifesaving. Worldwide, vaccinations have led to the near eradication of many dreaded illnesses like polio, typhoid, tetanus, etc. They protect many who otherwise would get sick from diseases like HIV and Ebola. Smallpox is the only disease completely eradicated by vaccines, and many infections are coming back because people have stopped getting vaccinations.

Unfortunately, only about 70% of children in the U.S. today receive routine vaccinations because many parents have become afraid the vaccine may cause autism or something worse. In recent years, the number of unvaccinated youths has led to a measles outbreak at Disney World and is currently in Texas and New Mexico. Most who resist protecting their children with routine vaccinations are affluent, educated white people. Alas, education is no protection against fear and unwise decisions.

Discovering Functional Medicine

Even today, as information about alternative and complementary therapies is becoming increasingly widespread, natural therapies are still being discounted because they haven't been "scientifically proven"—that is, been through a double-blind controlled study. Part of this is because natural therapies do not make money for large pharmaceutical companies, so who will pay to study them? In addition, they often involve more than one factor, which is hard to control in a double-blind study.

During my search for an effective anti-inflammatory diet, I ran across Dr. Dale Bredesen's book, *The End of Alzheimer's*. A practitioner of functional medicine,[53] Dr. Bredesen has been able to successfully treat up to 90% of his patients with memory problems, including some patients with the APOE4 gene found in Alzheimer's disease.

When I tried to find out why his approach had not been universally embraced by those in the medical profession treating memory problems, I was told, "Because this method has not been scientifically proven." It turns out there were too many variables involved in doing a placebo-controlled trial!

Dr. Bredesen takes a functional medicine approach based on identifying the cause of a problem, not just giving medications to control symptoms—the standard approach of American medicine. Functional medicine physicians evaluate inflammatory, metabolic, toxic, and nutritional conditions that can give rise to memory problems or make them worse. Then, they address these findings.

Inflammation may be caused by an infection, injury, or autoimmune disorder, in which the patient's immune system mistakenly attacks healthy tissue. Metabolic disorders include chemical changes like those seen in diabetes or gout. Toxic causes of memory problems include lead and mercury exposure as well as long-term exposure to irritants, such as industrial chemicals or polluted air.

Nutritional deficiencies can involve various substances, including vitamins, especially vitamin D. Recently, researchers have found that low vitamin D can create problems for people with multiple sclerosis and many other chronic conditions. Allopathic doctors evaluate some of these factors when assessing people who present with memory difficulties, but not in such detail.

Today, more people are turning to alternative and complementary

53   Functional medicine is aimed at finding the root cause of disease by identifying the nutritional, toxic, metabolic, and inflammatory causes of a disease.

medicine for help. Forty percent of Americans use some form of alternative or complementary medicine, even though they must pay out-of-pocket for it. Many mainstream hospitals include alternative and complementary therapies in day spas at their facilities.

Allopathic medical criticism of other therapies is also becoming less effective since so much of modern medicine is toxic to the human body. I hear warnings about natural therapies that the FDA hasn't studied, but we tend to forget that natural therapies are generally safe and do not cause harm, whereas too many FDA-approved medicines and procedures have the potential to cause injury and even death.

Remember, the third leading cause of death in the U.S. is medical error, but the fourth leading cause of death is from prescribed FDA-approved medical treatment. One year, during a doctor's strike in Canada, the death rate actually went down.

There are plenty of good books on exercise and diet, and the internet is available to anyone who wants to explore any avenue of movement and eating. But the standard medical establishment is still calling the shots, consuming all the money and political energy.

There is still debate about whether poor people deserve to be insured in our modern medical circus. That's because doctors oppose universal health insurance so they can make more money. And now we have businessman-owned hospitals and medical practices that target what is offered to make money. No one seems to care that making money drives the medical care we receive rather than what is best for our health.

It seems to me that the resistance to focusing on prevention and safer, less toxic therapies goes back to medicine's war on natural therapies, which has always been a competition for power and money. This moment in medicine reminds me of my first encounter with orthomolecular psychiatrists over fifty years ago, when I saw how much better patients with schizophrenia were when they received interventions to encourage good health and stable lives.

The good news is that alternative therapies are working their way back into American healthcare. Although about 40% of Americans use alternative therapies, this still makes alternative medicine outside the mainstream, thanks to our mental blind spot fostered by the medical profession.

Even in the political arena, while politicians call for universal healthcare and the end of private insurance and the influence of insurance money on the practice of medicine, we do not yet hear a call to rethink how the whole healthcare system operates or to ban advertising and focus on making money rather than making healthcare more focused on healing.

The American healthcare system should cover screenings, prevention programs for drug use and abuse, mental health, nutrition, physical therapy, and even birth control and protection for safe sex. The Affordable Care Act (ACA) tried to address some of these issues, but it has been fiercely resisted by those who want to support the financial basis of medicine, making money, and not encouraging better health for the American public in general.

But there is more. Unless we find a way to structure our approach to care to include tracking patients over a lifetime and using specialty care only for operations or other specialized treatments, we will not be able to break the cycle of over-testing and failure to address the needs of particular patients at particular times in their lives.

In the British Isles, everyone has a nurse practitioner who follows their care and doctors who focus on specialty interventions. It's a way to ensure everyone gets consistent care while getting the high-tech interventions when they are needed. Today's medical care is like my days at County Hospital when patients with chronic pain got the care they needed, including attention to depression and other psychiatric issues, on an ongoing basis in our clinic, and were sent to specialty doctors in their clinics only when they needed those specific services.

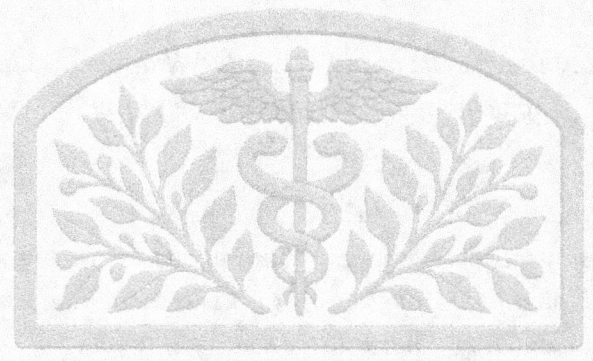

PART THREE

THE MISUSE OF SCIENCE

How modern medicine feeds the opiate epidemic, and finally, the problems with modern medicine exposed by the Covid pandemic and what we must do about it.

"What misery to be afraid of death. What wretchedness, to believe only in what can be proven."
— MARY OLIVER

"What happens then is like what when we separate a jigsaw puzzle into its five hundred pieces: The over-all picture disappears. This is the state of modern medicine: It has lost the sense of the unity of man. Such is the price it has paid for its scientific progress. It has sacrificed art to science."
— PAUL TOURNIER

"I am not against all forms of high-tech medicine. Drugs and surgeries have a secure place in the treatment of serious health conditions. But modern American medicine treats almost every health condition as if it were an emergency."
— ANDREW WEIL

How Using Science as the Only Standard to Understand the Patient is Limiting What Doctors Have to Offer

Doctors have always struggled to do what is best for their patients, but too often, their therapies are dangerous or toxic, making people worse or even killing them. Even today, the third and fourth leading causes of death are medical error[54] and treatment,[55] that is—standard medical treatment. (Cancer and heart disease are the first and second leaders of causes of death in the U.S.) So, the medical profession was inspired to adopt so-called evidence-based medicine (EBM)[56] to correct errors in the practice of medicine.

54 N.I.H. Recent studies of medical errors for as many as 251,000 deaths annually in the US, making medical errors the third leading cause of death.

55 N.I.H. Death from medical treatment (and errors, I presume) could be as high as 440,000 per year. Other statistics worth noting include unnecessary surgery, which is believed to cause about 12,000 deaths each year. More than 100,000 deaths each year might be related to medication complications.

56 The term EBM is relatively new. Investigators at McMaster University in Canada

Prior to this time, doctors used lab data and other information to help them with their deliberations, but data was only one factor in deciding what course to take with a particular patient. In 1996, the term was more formally defined by Sacket et al., who stated that EBM was "the conscientious and judicious use of current best evidence from clinical care research in the management of individual patients." Add to that the focus on business initiated by the ruling by the FDA on advertising in medicine, and we face a dangerous situation.

Understanding How Bias Affects Decision-Making

THERE ARE NUMEROUS WAYS errors and bias can slip into interactions between patients and doctors trying to apply the latest scientific advice to treat their patients.

First, the science itself may be flawed. From my earliest experience as a research fellow in 1965, I observed how errors can totally negate study results. Thanks to my first research experience, I learned never to accept anyone else's data without checking everything myself. Even then, I would have missed errors in the research lab concerning machines and equipment. The lab director told us, "What counts is what's in print." But that doesn't mean what's in print is always accurate or true.

I found errors everywhere, from the design of the study using middle-aged men as a control for pregnant women to errors in the build of the machines using twice as much pressure as indicated, and errors in how the material was being entered into the computers.

In addition, I observed the lab director telling grant providers what they wanted to hear rather than the literal truth, which indicates

began using the term during the 1990s. EBM was first defined as "a systemic approach to analyze published research as the basis of clinical decision making.

that lying or false representation is part of the research process at all levels.

Most research is funded by agencies or groups that want to prove a particular point or push a particular agenda. For example, when people from the food industry staff the FDA, FDA-funded studies will be carried out to prove items beneficial to the food industry instead of items aimed at the nation's best health. Experiments will be skewed by their original intent.

Perhaps the biggest problem with the science here is inherent in the placebo-controlled trial itself. The goal of such a trial is to prove that Substance X is more effective than a sugar pill administered by an enthusiastic clinician. That approach acknowledges even sugar pills presented by a clinician may have some healing or therapeutic effects, but it completely ignores the fact that natural therapies have been treating the condition in question for centuries without toxic side effects. Nowhere does it compare the effects of Substance X with these previously prescribed natural substances.

The use of inert substances as controls means a potentially toxic drug is not being compared with a probably much safer natural therapy. (Have you seen all those TV ads for medications with warnings about the possibility of dangerous side effects, including death?)

Furthermore, this much safer natural therapy is maybe one that organized medicine has been trying to discredit for over one hundred years because it represents competition. (See chapters on Rockefeller and the AMA.)

In addition, most drug trials are set up by drug companies to evaluate a new medication, procedure, or intervention in which they have a financial interest. As a result, studies are set up to present their product in the most favorable light. No one is studying things in which there is no financial interest.

What's more, researchers—like all humans—have egos that may lead them to inflate their successes or try to discredit their rivals. This process may undoubtedly delay, if not distort, the facts.

The national response to AIDS research and tracking is a particularly egregious example. While homophobia may have affected those at the National Institutes of Health (NIH) who failed to fund the tracking of the disease nationally or invest in substantial research into the cause and treatment of AIDS, prominent researchers at NIH still attempted to thwart French researchers and steal their claims of being the first to find the cause of the disease.[57]

How Science Has Changed Our Understanding of the World

AS A CULTURE, WE have bought into the scientific mantle that "statistics" are used to "prove" things, and that the veil of statistics has so overtaken our way of thinking, it has invaded the lexicon.

Just as noble and base once reflected the "nobility" and "baser" elements in society, so too were "normal" and "deviant" once statistical terms. The problem is that normal and deviant have become more than descriptors of what is. They now define the basis for evaluating behavior, for accepting or rejecting a standard.

One has only to watch daytime television to see how acceptable "normal" behavior has become. As a standard for "good and bad" in our society—it's now "normal" for college students to cheat and corporation executives to loot their companies and politicians to be beholden to their financial backers, just as it's normal for physicians to focus on the business of their practice and see patients as potential adversaries.

57   See "And the Band Played ON".

The threat of a lawsuit has always driven the use of technology in this country, dating back to the introduction of X-ray machines in the early 20th century. In this country, lawsuits are settled by juries rather than by an official board, as in other countries.

But there was a time when suits were much rarer. That was a time when physicians donated their time to those who couldn't pay. Lawyers like Clarence Darrow stood for what was right, not just what he was paid for, and how much money they could make. That which was wrong was not glorified because it made lots of money.

A society dominated by science and money is a valueless society, as demonstrated by Richard Dawkins in *The Selfish Gene*. Without value and standards, selfishness is built into our genes.

Our wars are now high-tech fiascos like our high-tech medicine because they don't address meaning. We are currently horrified at all the civilian casualties in Gaza, but when we were killing in Iraq and Afghanistan, we suppressed the number of dead that resulted from our own bombing. Both war and science have become other means of acting out and making the most money.

Cutting the Patient's Input Out of Decision Making Makes Medicine Super Expensive and Too Often Irrelevant and Dangerous

The attempt to standardize medical treatment is laudable; however, as history has shown us, evidence and data do not always translate into the best application of medical decisions and treatment. Medical decisions and policies should be based on science to ensure doctors provide the best treatment and prevent them from harming their patients as much as possible. However, practicing medicine involves more than just assessing data. It involves understanding the patient with the disease and responding to that patient's needs and fears. Too often, by just ordering tests, a doctor will miss the best intervention for that particular patient at that particular moment, which may not involve life-threatening medications, procedures, or surgery.

This point becomes more critical when the focus is more on making money. As a result, doctors spend less time with their patients and tend to trust tests more than the patients and their information.

Having passed 80 years old, I was delighted to hear that if I got COVID, I would not be put on a ventilator. Most people who spend much time on a ventilator develop multiple physical and mental problems, so they may not be dead, but their quality of life may be nil. Quality of life does not seem to be part of the equation anymore. Only what earns money and what avoids a lawsuit.

Alas, when medical decisions are driven by tests and money rather than wisdom and judgment, patients will get all kinds of medical evaluations and procedures because someone is ready to do them, not because that is in that patient's best interest. That will ensure that too much harmful therapy still gets through.

Evidence-based medicine was introduced to standardize medical practice based on the latest peer-reviewed studies. Unfortunately, information sometimes gets to the public before the definitive study has been completed or while doctors are still trying to determine the validity of a published study. So, in spite of EBM, doctors can still be behind the times or operate on information before it has been verified.

Shortly after my husband's heart procedure to put in stents, data appeared condemning the practice. When they catheterized my husband the following year to look at the stents, they found the vessels with the stents had collapsed, so the stents were not doing him any good. By then, he had already been through three potentially dangerous procedures for naught. EBM was designed to prevent unnecessary procedures, but its application has been imperfect, like all human endeavors.

To close the gap between what is best for a particular patient at a particular time and what tests and procedures the doctor offers, it's essential to realize that one cannot always use test data to evaluate what will lead to healing. Since scientific studies have shown that patients respond to what they believe about themselves more than to what tests show,[58] The body's capacity for healing is more complicated and complex than we currently know or understand.

There is another reason why testing may not be the best approach for helping patients. Human beings make decisions based on emotion, not facts. Let me say that again: humans make decisions based on emotion, not facts.

In medicine, if we only trust information gleaned from tests and physical exams, we too often fail to use the emotional connection in the doctor-patient relationship to explore the patient's concerns which could lead to a better understanding of this particular patient at this particular time and thus lead to a more constructive treatment plan and positive self-healing attitude. Also, this is when patients might reveal their suicidal thoughts or despair about the future.

The weakness in my legs after four rounds of antibiotics in 2014 is a case in point. My plan has always been to exercise every day. Even if I'm sick, I generally get up and exercise and stretch a little. Then, I go back to bed for the day. The longer I'm sick or the more often I'm sick, the less and less I exercise. When that happens, I'll get so weak I have to start at the beginning of my exercise routine and gradually build up to regain my strength. There is no test I

58   In one study, patients were given the opposite report of what their tests showed. In general, these patients' outcomes matched what they believed about themselves and their health, rather than what their test results had shown.

know that will identify infections and a lack of exercise as the cause of increased weakness. I was fully aware this was the cause of my weakness and would have shared this fact if anyone had given me the chance.

But when I went to see the neurologist, he wanted to run tests on the basis of his resident's exam. He never even took a history from me about why I might be weaker. A physician should be trained to delve into these kinds of facts and sort out the problem rather than merely run tests that tell him whether I'm having an MS flare, or my spinal cord is being impinged upon.

I have not been as savvy about food as I have been about exercise. I could have used the help of a doctor who was curious and knowledgeable enough to help me figure out that eating sweets and certain other foods might be weakening my immune system. Instead, the perverse approach of ordering tests first and asking questions later—or not at all—has never been helpful to me.

Valuing information gleaned from a test over the patient's history or experience makes medicine much more expensive and robs the patient of a chance to have their problem unraveled and solved on the spot by a caring physician. Instead, they're forced to wait anxiously for test results. If the test isn't helpful, the doctor will often shrug and give up as if he has done his job!

The excuse for not talking with patients is often a lack of time, which is too often demanded by business-oriented practices out to make the most money. But even when doctors do spend time talking with patients, they no longer see their role as problem-solvers. Instead, they see their function as ordering tests and writing prescriptions.

The medical system today has become so standardized to

diagnose or rule out grave illnesses or conditions that respond to pills, shots, procedures, or surgery that doctors have lost the art of unraveling the problems that bring patients to the doctor in the first place.

I am managing my MS well, but for me, being weaker or unable to do as much exercise is very serious. Problem-solving conversations, not tests, are what I need from time to time.

The Importance of the Doctor-Patient Relationship and Empathy to the Safety of the Patient

THIS INVESTIGATIVE STANCE, GROUNDED in EBM, stands apart from the doctor's role in promoting the placebo effect or encouraging healing. For the placebo effect to work, the patient must believe in their doctor and their treatment, mostly through the vehicle of the doctor-patient relationship. This is an intimate relationship that takes time to develop. In recent times, when a doctor you do not know sees you in an emergency situation or when you are hospitalized, we lose the benefit of that relationship to care for patients.

In recent years, when I noticed myself getting depressed, I asked for help and was sent to a psychologist who worked with MS patients. I thought this might be useful to have someone who could understand my struggles with MS. Her approach involved getting patients to take some action to solve their problems. Since I was already taking action, she was not much help. What I really needed was someone who could explore what was troubling me. We may feel sad or frustrated, but not be fully aware of what is bothering us. That's when a skilled interviewer is most helpful in getting to the core of the problem.

I remember one young man with cancer coming to consult me.

"I'm so glad to be seeing someone who wants to know more about me than whether I've found any new lumps and if I'm still throwing up," he said.

I thought to myself that most of the time, I only wanted to know in my outpatient clinic if patients had been hearing voices or not sleeping at night. These were issues I could address with medication, but I was also aware of how to get patients to give me more information when that was important.

It's not that I did not use checklists to cover other extraneous issues, but I did know when to look further and probe deeper. I knew focusing on their behavior and emotions was the key to understanding my patients. These are the signs I needed to dig deeper. In my experience, doctors too often assume they know why a patient is anxious, irritable, depressed, or acting out rather than take the time to ask and find out the real cause of their behavior.

Even physicians who talk about having empathy or sympathy for patients are still much too focused on themselves and their own emotions. They're concentrating on how they feel, not the patient's feelings. It's natural and unavoidable for a doctor to experience various emotions when dealing with different medical situations.

The critical point here is that if physicians are to understand what's happening with the patient, the doctor must explore changes in the patient's behavior and all expressions of emotion, including pseudo-neurologic symptoms. These alarm bells tell doctors to spend more time with the patient, listening and figuring out what is going on by responding to what they actually see and hear.

It may also be appropriate to complete a structured mental status exam with the patient to be sure they are not suffering from mental confusion or delirium caused by medication or disease.

I will never forget one patient with multiple sclerosis I was asked to see in the hospital. She was instructed to get up and walk around, but the doctors kept finding her lying flat in bed.

After seeing her, I realized she was too confused to follow instructions. Testing revealed her oxygen level was so low that she could not follow through with anything. There is definitely a place for ordering tests, but it helps to delve into what the patient is experiencing so we can at least order the proper tests!

When asking about a patient's feelings and behavior, physicians don't have to be correct in their interpretations of what is going on. Patients will correct their mistakes—so long as doctors give the patient a chance to speak. Here is an example.

Doctor: "You must be feeling overwhelmed with having to manage a full-time job while you're dealing with MS."

Patient: "No, I'm pissed off because I've been trying to get a referral to physical therapy for two months and can't get anyone to respond."

Too often, physicians are focused on their own agendas or feelings. They may tell funny stories due to their own discomfort or, nowadays, are too focused on their computer screen to really hear what the patient is saying. Exploring a patient's emotions and/or behavior isn't time-consuming, but it does require knowing when to pay attention and focus on what has changed.

"We as a profession have caused an epidemic that is bigger than the HIV epidemic. We have more deaths from drug overdoses than occurred at the peak of the HIV/AIDS epidemic in 1995. That's how big this is. It's more deaths than in motor vehicle accidents. The cause in the opioid epidemic starts with getting a prescription of opioids from physicians."
— A. Gawande MD

"Habit is habit, and not to be flung out of the window by any man, but coaxed downstairs a step at a time."
— Mark Twain

The Opiate Epidemic: Are Doctors Making Us Worse? This is What You Need to Know to Assess and Safely Treat Chronic Pain

In 2012, well-trained by the medical profession and the pharmaceutical companies, Americans consumed 80% of the world's pain medicines or opiates. Alabama became number one in the nation in the number of opiate prescriptions.

That was the year I published two books about chronic pain, depression, and addiction. I had been working with patients who had depression and chronic pain, many of them addicts.

In the process, I realized that not only did the patients not know what to do, but neither did too many of their physicians. Some doctors were passing out too many opiate prescriptions without offering anything else. But some doctors refused to give opiates at all because they thought too many abused the drugs.

No doctors I saw were using opiates to improve function rather than just make patients feel better. Functioning in all its myriad ways helps us get well, so using opiates should be aimed at improved function.

In 2017, I was admitted to the hospital with a blood infection (sepsis). Every day, I was shocked at how the practice of medicine had changed in ten years since I retired. During my stay, I never once saw a doctor who knew me. Today, doctors called "hospitalists" treat patients in the hospital. I presume that if you have something like cancer and need several admissions, you will see the same doctors or medical team each time you go to the hospital, but for a one-off problem like sepsis, there was no one involved in my care who knew anything about me. The doctor did not even make rounds to see me until late in the day.

In addition to not having a doctor I could rely on during that hospital stay, I observed several dangerous practices for patients, including several lost opportunities to educate patients about self-care. One of the most glaring flaws was in pain management.

Day and night, every few hours, a bright young nurse came by to ask me to rate my pain level from one to ten. I hadn't been admitted because of pain, and she did not inquire about any specific pain or where my pain might be located; she just wanted a number for my pain between one and ten to put on a man chart.

Assessing pain in this way is called the "fifth vital sign," which is recorded at a clinic visit or every few hours in the hospital along with the other vital signs: pulse rate, blood pressure, respiration, and temperature, all of which can be measured directly. Even though the pain experience is subjective and not something nurses can measure, pain was added as the fifth vital sign in the mid-1990s in an attempt to alert doctors when a patient's pain needed to be reevaluated. Knowing this, I eventually decided to speak up. "

Do you mean the pain in my head, the pain in my abdomen, or the pain in my big toe?" I had slid down into the bed, and my toe was killing me.

The poor young nurse couldn't tell me. Apparently, no one was watching to see if my abdominal pain was getting worse.

Because I had run a pain clinic, I knew the pain scale she was using was supposed to trigger an assessment if I answered seven or higher. I also knew that in practice, an answer of seven or higher routinely triggered staff to provide more pain medicines, even opiates, and did not lead to a new assessment.

Apparently, the act of asking a patient to rate their pain 1-10 was considered the pain assessment! Rather than looking into what might be making the pain worse, doctors would simply give the patient more pain medicine, even if the medicine itself could be causing the increased pain.

Pain medications can lead to increased pain during the withdrawal period, when the effect of the pain medicine is wearing off, so doctors who are treating withdrawal pain with more medicine may create a never-ending cycle.

What You Need to Know About Assessment

WHY IS AN ASSESSMENT important? First of all, 80% of chronic pain is musculoskeletal. That means, even in cancer patients with pain from metastases in their bones, inactivity may increase their pain from tight muscles and tendons, and they need to move and stretch to lessen this pain. Just taking more and more opiates does not solve that problem.

Another reason assessment is essential is that opiates and other pain meds may cause increased pain or rebound pain and may make the pain worse. When neurosurgeons first decided to insert a stimulator into the brain itself to relieve intractable pain, they first took their patients off all pain meds to assess their actual level of baseline pain before the procedure. Eighty percent of these patients became pain-free after six weeks, even patients who were addicted to their drugs! Even addicts![59]

Daily opiate use is a major cause of chronic pain. Eighteen months after an injury, all opiates and other pain meds need to be stopped because healing is complete by that time, and most will not need any daily pain meds. Old injuries can act up from time to time, so periodic opiates to manage function may still make sense.

I used to have daily migraine headaches and took one Excedrin Migraine every morning. I stopped that pill after I got a stomach ulcer, and my morning headaches went away altogether. So, all pain medications, as well as coffee and other substances, can cause rebound pain. Beware! Watch everything you ingest regularly if you have chronic headaches.

Comprehensive Pain Assessment

A COMPREHENSIVE PAIN ASSESSMENT means stepping back and considering whether the present approach to managing pain is working. It means first evaluating what's causing the pain.

Is it nerve pain, which is burning, shooting, or tingling like

---

59   Anyone who takes opiates daily will develop tolerance to the effects of the opiate, needing to take larger and larger doses over time to have the same effect. That is not addiction. Addiction results when the individual continues to take the medicine in spite of evidence of negative effects of the drug.

electricity, or muscle pain, which tends to be dull, aching, or throbbing? Visceral or internal pains tend to be cramping, distending, or squeezing.

Secondly, doctors should assess where the pain is located. Some pains are localized at the problem area, while others appear in other parts of the body, such as heart pain in the right arm or neck. Thirdly, doctors must consider how the pain has changed, including what makes it better and what makes it worse.

Next, they need to examine what the patient has tried to alleviate the pain, such as movement, stretching, distraction, or medicines. Finally, depression must be looked for in anyone suffering from chronic pain since 75% of those with chronic pain have depression, which benefits from being treated with daily exercise and antidepressant medication.

Then There is Inactivity

ANY CAUSE OF PAIN, even pain from cancer, may be made worse by inactivity, so movement, stretching, and massage may lessen that pain as well. Patients with cancer pain may hurt more when they're afraid the pain means their cancer is spreading.

So, everyone should have strategies other than medications to deal with anxiety. This can include movement, listening to music, relaxation exercises, massage, meditation, self-hypnosis, and many other techniques.

But they should also have an opportunity to express their concerns. Even diet can affect pain. Some people cannot eat meat, while others are affected by nightshade vegetables (tomatoes, peppers, eggplant, and potatoes).

In addition, different types of pain respond best to different types of medicines. Thus, thoroughly investigating a patient's medicines and their side effects is an important part of a pain assessment. Of course, worsening pain needs to be assessed for other reasons. Sometimes, increasing pain means a problem is spreading or, worse, requires an intervention like surgery.

Sometimes, talking it out with a caring person may be more helpful than anything. And sometimes, worsening pain just means the patient has been sitting too long in one position or has slid down in bed and needs to get up, move around, and stretch.

The failure to see pain assessments in these terms is a major contributor to the opiate crisis in this country. For that reason and other problems, defining pain assessment as the fifth vital sign was removed by the Joint Commission governing hospitals in 2016. However, that did not stop the process because physicians are not taught about all aspects of pain and pain intervention.

Focusing on Pain Makes It Worse and Sends the Wrong Message

BACK IN THE HOSPITAL, nurses were getting patients to focus on their pain level every few hours, which always makes pain worse because distraction is a major way to treat pain, instead of training patients to associate hurting with taking more medicine. Likewise, doctors were training patients to take pills rather than teaching them to do all the other activities that mitigate pain.

Distraction is a Major Way to Manage Pain

ONE OF MY PROFESSORS told this story. He got a scratch in his eye and went to the ER. They looked at his eye with a slit lamp and said it was just a scratch and would heal in a few days. The next day, he went to work and did fine until he came home and sat in his comfy chair. Then his eye started hurting again. It hurt so much that he went back to the ER. The ER doctors said it looked fine and would heal in a few days.

The next day, he was pain-free all day until he came home and sat in his chair. Only then did his eye hurt and feel as bad as before. This time, he finally realized what was happening. As long as he was busy and focused elsewhere, he did not hurt. Only when he was no longer busy did he feel how much the eye hurt him.

Since distraction is a critical way to manage pain, asking a patient to focus minutely on their pain to rate it from 1-10 can actually make the pain appear worse. And just giving patients pills in response to more pain trains them to seek out pills first, instead of last, when they hurt. It does not encourage using distraction, movement, or relaxation to get better instead.

Since no pain medicine is 100% effective anyway, it behooves us all to have a range of strategies to help manage periodic or worsening pain which is part of everyone's life. Even at night, when pain is always worse, it's wise to have activities or topics to think about as you fall asleep. It does not have to be counting sheep!

Distraction and movement are major ways we deal with pain. What a lost opportunity in the hospital to train patients how to manage their pain rather than take pain pills! What if the nurses, when they came around, had gotten me to stand up and do a few stretches, walk up and down the hall, or taught me how to self-massage, soothe myself with music, or distract myself with other mental or physical activities?

Since older people may hurt more than young people because they are more often idle, getting patients to focus on how much they hurt and take pills, the medical profession is encouraging behavior that can not only lead to more pain and drug-drug interactions in their patients, but may even promote addiction as well!

It's time for a thoughtful change. It's time to teach activities that would actually help you manage, including exercise and meditation, dietary changes, and returning to a normal routine.

Opiates Should Be Used to Improve Function

ANOTHER PROBLEM IS WHEN doctors give prescriptions for opiates that say, "as needed for pain," they are not training the patient to take the medicine to improve function, rather than just to "feel" better. Taking medicine to get dressed in the morning, if that is hard, before exercising, so they can get through their morning routine or interact with others, is taking medicine to improve function. Doctors should not be prescribing opiates so patients feel better, but so they can do better and function better.

A Place for Opiate Management

OPIATES CAN BE LIFESAVING in managing the pain of heart attacks, sickle cell crises, or severe burns, where pain can be a killer. Opiates are helpful in controlling post-op pain for many patients so they can get going again. Opiates are even helpful in managing chronic pain if used to maximize function, to be more active, socialize, and have sex.

Too often, doctors just write "tid prn" (three times a day as needed for pain) on the prescription, or more recently, every eight hours, rather than tying the use of the medication to increased activity or involvement with others. Since these medicines don't last eight hours, many wear off after three hours, which can be very misleading. I have met many fine doctors over the years who were blind to the effects of their opiate-prescribing practices.

At the same time, opioid overdose can be life-threatening. If you take opiates with other medicines or substances that affect the central nervous system, like alcohol, tranquilizers, or sleeping pills, you have an increased chance of having breathing problems or even death.

What a wasted opportunity for patient education! I thought at the time. If each of these pain visits had included questions about how often I'd been moving around in bed, instructions on how to do bed exercises, or simple exercises like walking down the hall or going to the bathroom, they could have been helpful education tools for pain management.

Movement is important throughout life, and people who are sick or have chronic illnesses are less likely to exercise or even move. They could be taught how to constantly make little movements, stretching their muscles and tendons. Little movements in bed or when they are sitting or walking to the bathroom would help with pain management, which is often brought on by inactivity, and also help older people learn the best way to stay supple and pain-free for life. Hospital settings and routines would be a natural place for this kind of education.

The nurses might even return to giving patients massages, which will help them a lot more than being asked over and over to rate their pain level! Given what we now know about the opiate epidemic in America, it should be considered malpractice to continue such practices, but it fits perfectly with the Big Pharma takeover of medicine and the war against natural therapies I have observed throughout my medical career.

This practice of giving pills for pain is so widespread and so much a part of the standard American medical practice that I'm afraid no one will want to make a change. Doctors and hospitals make money passing out pills and treating conditions caused by the

American diet and lifestyle. Training patients to exercise and eat anti-inflammatory diets would work against the American medical industry.

In my case, because I kept eating sweets, ice cream, and other such things both in and after I left the hospital, I spent the following summer having stomach issues. That fall, I went from one infection to another until I went back on an anti-inflammatory diet two weeks before Christmas.

It took my GI tract six months to recover completely from taking four antibiotics in the hospital. Fortunately, the fall infections were common viruses, so I did not even think about calling my doctor except to refill my steroid inhaler, which I'd used in the past for wheezing when I got viral pneumonia.

Training everyone to focus on their pain level and tying it to taking pills encourages more and more pill-taking. So, using pain as the fifth vital sign is facilitating the opiate epidemic. Prescribing stronger and stronger opiates like OxyContin has also contributed to this issue.

Since the early 1990s, doctors have been prescribing many more opioid painkillers such as codeine, hydrocodone, morphine, and oxycodone, supposedly because more people are living with chronic pain. But doctors are not well-trained to deal with pain or assess the pain they see. So, although they may not hand out as many opiates, they are not managing pain even after surgery well.

History of America's Approach to Drugs

MANY CURRENTLY ILLEGAL DRUGS, such as marijuana, opium, cocaine, and psychedelics, have been used for thousands of years for both medical and spiritual purposes. However, starting in the 19th century, states and municipalities began restricting certain drugs based on the communities that commonly used them rather than on any scientific assessment of risks.

The first American drug law was passed in San Francisco in 1875 and was directed at Chinese immigrants by banning the smoking of opium in opium dens. Anti-cocaine laws initiated in the early 1900s were directed at black men in the South. Anti-marijuana laws in the 1910s and 1920s were directed at Mexicans in the Southwest.

In the 1960s, street drugs became symbols of youthful rebellion along with protests against the Vietnam War. At the time, no one knew that the so-called "War on Drugs" begun by President Nixon in 1971, ostensibly to address the problem of addiction in this country, was actually a covert way to incarcerate anti-Vietnam War hippies and black people who presented a challenge for the president.

In America, government officials have been trying to criminalize drug use in minority populations since San Francisco initiated the anti-opium law in 1875, but Nixon was the first to do it for political purposes.

John Ehrlichman, Nixon's domestic policy advisor, told Mark Perry, who was interviewing him for an article for *The Atlantic* in April 2016, "You want to know what this was really all about? The Nixon Campaign in 1968 and the Nixon White House had two enemies: the anti-war left and black people. You understand what I am saying? We knew we could not make it illegal to be either against the war or being black, but by getting the public to associate the hippies with marijuana and blacks with heroin, and then criminalizing both heavily, we could disrupt those communities. We could arrest their leaders, raid their homes, break up their meetings, and vilify them night after night on the evening news. Did we know we were lying about the drugs? Of course, we did."

If there's any doubt that the War on Drugs started by Nixon

in the 1970s was a ploy to lock up black people, look at what it has accomplished since then. The incarceration rate of black males was stable at 200 per 100,000 for fifty years between 1920 and 1970.

That rate had doubled by 1986, quadrupled by 1996, and peaked at 956 per 100,000 in 2008. Yet at the same time, opiate deaths rose from about 7,000 per 100,000 in 1970 to more than 17,000 per 100,000 in 2019. Clearly, focusing on criminalizing drug use is not stopping drug use; it's only undermining the black community.[60]

In 1972, the Federal Drug Commission unanimously recommended decriminalizing the possession and distribution of marijuana for personal use. Nixon ignored the report and rejected its recommendations. Between 1973 and 1977, various states, along with Congress, moved to decriminalize marijuana possession. However, within just a few years, the tide had shifted, and proposals to decriminalize marijuana were abandoned. Marijuana was ultimately caught up in a broader cultural backlash against the permissiveness of the 1970s.

Public concern about illicit drug use built throughout the 1980s, mainly due to media portrayals of people addicted to the smoking form of cocaine, dubbed "crack." Soon after Ronald Reagan took office in 1981, his wife, Nancy Reagan, began a highly publicized anti-drug campaign, coining the slogan "Just say no."

This set the stage for the zero-tolerance drug policies implemented in the mid-to-late 1980s. Congress and state legislatures alike passed draconian penalties for drug possession and use that rapidly increased the prison population. Harsh drug policies also blocked

---

60   Every president since then has found the "war on drugs" useful. Reagan even used Panamanian dictator Manuel Noriega and the drug cartels to introduce cocaine into the black community in Los Angeles in order to more freely arrest blacks for drug use.

the expansion of syringe-access programs and other harm-reduction policies that could have reduced the rapid spread of HIV/AIDS.

It's important to note the role media hype played in public concern about America's drug problem. From a baseline of 6%, polls showed that public concern rose to 64% in the 1980s but dropped back to 10% after media attention waned.

Although Bill Clinton claimed to be in favor of treatment for dealing with drugs rather than incarceration, he continued to escalate the drug war once he was in office. He rejected federal funding for syringe-access programs as well as a U.S. Sentencing Commission recommendation to eliminate the disparity in sentences between crack cocaine used in the black community and powder cocaine used in the white communities.

In recent years, public opinion in the U.S. has shifted dramatically in favor of sensible reforms that expand health-based approaches to addiction while reducing the role of criminalization in drug policy. Reflecting this change in attitudes, then-President Obama supported several successful policy changes, such as reducing the crack/powder sentencing disparity, ending the ban on federal funding for syringe-access programs, and ending federal interference with state medical marijuana laws. However, he did not shift the majority of drug-policy funding to match the increasingly popular health-based approach.

The first Trump administration threatened to take us backward toward an 1980s-style drug war. President Trump vowed to build a wall on the U.S.-Mexico border to keep drugs out of the country and called for harsher sentences for drug-law violations and the death penalty for people who sell drugs. He also resurrected the ineffective "just say no" messaging aimed at youth.

Today, more and more states are legalizing marijuana, and

legalizing it nationally is more popular than ever. In 2013, Uruguay became the first country in the world to legally regulate marijuana. Canada legalized marijuana for adults in 2018. In 2020, Oregon voters passed Measure 110, the nation's first all-drug decriminalization measure. This and other moves around the country confirm a substantial shift in public support for treating drug use with health services rather than with criminalization and prison.

Despite these reforms, approximately 700,000 people are still arrested for marijuana offenses each year, and almost 500,000 people are still behind bars for nothing more than a drug-law violation. Black and Latino communities are still subject to a disproportionate number of drug-related arrests and convictions, even though drug use among white upper and middle-class people is just as high.

Even worse, as marijuana, in particular, is increasingly legalized around the country, wealthy investors in the marijuana market are poised to make legal millions for doing the same thing that generations of people of color have been arrested and locked up for.

Former President Biden said we need a "compassionate approach" to problematic drug use, reducing the role of criminalization and increasing access to treatment and harm-reduction services for people who need them. What measures President Trump's Executive Actions will enact is anybody's guess.

"*There is nothing on this earth more to be prized than true friendship.*"
— Thomas Aquinas

"*The only thing that really matters in life are your relationships to other people.*"
— George Vaillant

The Future of Medicine: Genuine Healthcare for America: How Racism Has Limited Healthcare and Education for Everyone

The COVID-19 pandemic exploded in February 2020, just as I began working on my final chapter about genuine healthcare and the future of medicine. Listening to reports coming out of China, I knew right away, being an old person with MS, I would have to sequester myself for two years or more until the virus passed or a vaccine made it relatively safe to enter the world again.

I also knew that no one would be interested in my lifetime of discoveries about medicine and healing while our doctors and nurses were the heroes on the frontlines of the pandemic, risking their lives without adequate protective equipment (PPE) to save lives and treat the dying.

Who would care about medicine's war against natural therapies, the placebo effect, and what I had unearthed about John D. Rockefeller's role in shaping the profession? Who would care about the unconscious defense mechanisms driving the pursuit of money and the focus on biomedicine to the exclusion of psychosocial aspects of medicine, and fail to provide reasonable medical care for us all? Who would care about the medical profession's routine failings when the need for doctors was so dire?

The Marvels of Modern-Day Medicine

IN SO MANY WAYS, the practice of medicine has come a long way since the last great pandemic, the Spanish Flu of 1918. The U.S. has made major contributions to that advance. We should not forget that less than one hundred and fifty years ago, some reputable doctors were performing brutal surgeries without anesthesia. Other respected doctors were bleeding their patients and using leeches as treatment. Still, other highly regarded doctors were handing out medicines loaded with mercury, lead, and arsenic. It seems doctors have always been purveyors of death as well as healing.

Advances in public health, medical technology, and medications in the past fifty years have led to a staggering increase in life expectancy of almost thirty years, at least until COVID hit. Much of this progress is related to advances in public health, such as improved sanitation, the campaign against smoking, the use of seat belts and designated drivers who don't drink, regular screenings for life-threatening illnesses, and vaccinations to halt epidemics of infectious diseases.

In some countries, strict gun regulation has even ended that source of violent death and serious injury. In the same way, strict public health measures adopted by all, along with contact tracing, have controlled pandemics in many countries.

Other advances include the progress in imaging technology for making diagnoses and understanding medical problems, the use of microsurgery and robotics, and more sophisticated anesthesia, antibiotics, and anti-viral therapy, all of which have given life to many with chronic diseases ranging from AIDS to cancer to heart disease.

Organ transplantation has extended many lives, and advanced dialysis allows people unsuitable for transplant to live for long periods of time. Physician specialization has reached its apogee.

In addition, the clinical use of gene therapy and stem cell therapy has revolutionized the treatment of some cancers and other formerly deadly diseases. The use of randomized controlled trials of medications and checklists to limit the use of dangerous medications and medical practices have increased the safety of surgery and medical treatment for many.

Recently, information technology has revolutionized the practice of medicine by making vast arrays of information available to doctors and other medical professionals. The spread of the modern hospice movement has greatly improved patients' comfort and well-being at the end of life. We—and by that, I mean economically prosperous people—truly live in a grand medical world.

But then, COVID-19 spread, and the whole country shut down. Some foreign countries succeeded in getting the virus under control. Many Asian countries did better initially because they had faced the threat of SARS in recent years and because their cultures value the whole nation's health over the individual's health.

New York City, Seattle, and California generally became the country's epicenters of the COVID-19 virus. There was a shortage of masks, protective equipment (PPE), and ventilators everywhere. There were fears that the medical system would become too overwhelmed to respond to the outbreak.

Then-president Donald Trump apparently knew the situation, but he didn't want to panic the stock market, so he remained upbeat in the face of bad news. He also refused to wear a mask—a mask being a fairly standard practice to avoid a respiratory disease—to protect himself and those around him.

Trump went further, casting the wearing of masks and the closing of schools and offices to control the virus as political symbols of defeat. He even touted not following CDC guidelines as a symbol of independence. For some people, even protesting public health measures with assault weapons became acceptable.

A society that celebrates the rights of the individual over the rights of the community sacrifices certain protective measures in a medical crisis. In Alabama, some school officials, public health officers, and their families were threatened with violence for wanting to initiate public health measures to protect children in school.

Nationally, our public health system—once touted as the best in the world—failed to step up and fill the void left by the president. This defeat was reminiscent of the public health response to the AIDS epidemic years earlier, when prejudice against gay men led to a failure to study and respond to a raging plague. The shortfall in AIDS response was blamed on a lack of money and political interference from the president, then Ronald Reagan.

Regardless of the cause, the response to COVID exposed a public health system not focused on the health of the nation as a whole.

Then, citizens began dying—twice as many African Americans as Caucasians. The systemic racism in our healthcare system, which goes back centuries, has emerged from the shadows. The failure of predominantly Southern states to expand Medicaid even in the face of this COVID crisis demonstrated how glaring systemic racism still is to this day, especially in providing good medical care.

So, how are systemic racism and a healthcare system focused on making money rather than promoting health linked? To see the connection, we have to go back to the founding of this country.

Europeans came to these shores for centuries to gain riches from land, cheap labor, and abundant natural resources. From the beginning, wealth was based on African slavery and the brutality required to keep slaves in their place, plus the acquisition of new slaves and land from indigenous populations.

Africans and Native Americans were seen as less than human with the blessing of the Roman Catholic Church, which said they, like other animals, lacked a soul, justifying their enslavement. Unfortunately, the tendency to justify and rationalize horrendous behavior to demonize and brutalize Africans and native peoples, as ordained by God, continues today.

Accepting patients based on whether they can pay for healthcare and even brutalizing the poor to make a profit is nothing new. And thanks to decades of policies aimed at keeping blacks and Native Americans poor, these groups are the ones most often sidelined in our current medical system. Are we really willing to continue this behavior and say, "It's just the American way?"

In a September 2021 article in the *New York Times*, Nicholas Kristof[61] made a stunning indictment of our system. In spite of immense wealth, military power, and cultural influence, the United States ranks twenty-eighth in the world on the Social Progress Scale in quality of life and health.

This index measures fifty aspects of well-being, including nutrition, health, education, safety, freedom, sanitation, environment, and more. According to Kristof, the United States is number one in the quality of our universities but ninety-first in access to quality basic education.

The U.S. is the best in the world in medical technology, but 97th

61   Nicholas Kristof, NYTimes, "We're No. 28 and dropping!", September 10, 2020.

in providing access to quality healthcare. Our health statistics are similar to those of Chile, Albania, and Jordan, while our citizens' education is on par with Uzbekistan and Mongolia.

Kristof went on to quote the Index director, Michael Green, "Societies that are tolerant, inclusive and better educated, are better able to manage the pandemic."

The Failures of Public Health . . . and What to Do About It

So now, we can clearly see the problem. In the last century, the medical profession has shifted its focus from what is in the best interest of patients to what makes the most money for doctors, hospitals, insurance companies, drug companies, and other peripheral medical services. This has, in turn, led to a shift in focus from what is best for the nation's health to a highly specialized, high-tech practice of medicine based on the market.

For decades, public health offerings have been increasingly defunded, and the focus on primary care and prevention activities has been greatly reduced, even though these interventions help us live longer and healthier lives. How did this happen?

In the 1980s, a number of malpractice suits led doctors to become very anxious about being sued. Suddenly, doctors shifted their focus from patient care to protecting themselves from a malpractice charge. Around the same time, the federal government cut Medicare payments to doctors.

I saw the result in the doctor's lounge. There was a shift from discussing what was wrong with patients and what was best for them to discussing practice issues and risk management. Doctors began seeing patients as potential adversaries.

Meanwhile, having patients interact more with staff than with doctors weakened the doctor-patient bond and weakened that health benefit, making patients more likely to sue and setting up a vicious cycle.

Practicing defensive medicine meant depending on lawyers more and the relationship with the patient less. I remember a time when doctors wept with their patients' families when something bad happened. Now, the doctor might not know the patient well enough to feel sad or care about the family.

Recently, my husband had a procedure. He was sent home with an opiate prescription to be filled and twenty pages of instructions. Somewhere in that ream of paper, it said to drink two glasses of water right away. However, since his pain was inadequately managed, he was too sick to his stomach to drink anything and ended up in the ER that night.

Even his opiate prescription was inadequate. It said to take one tablet every six hours for pain three times a day. But that type of pain medicine wears off after three hours and should be given more often in the first twenty-four hours when there is a great deal of pain. That experience clearly showed me how everyone is in trouble in today's medical world.

This trend in defunding public health and focusing on making money for doctors rather than providing the best care for patients ensured that the nation was not prepared to handle COVID when it arrived, nor will we be prepared when the next pandemic arrives. Hospitals did not have enough supplies on hand and could not cooperate with competing hospitals. Doctors and nurses were overwhelmed.

Focusing on health insurance, some U.S. presidents have proposed universal healthcare for over one hundred years, but the American Medical Society (AMA), representing organized medicine, medical insurance companies, and pharmaceutical companies, has opposed universal healthcare because doctors and drug companies won't make as much money under such a system. As it is, many doctors won't take new patients with Medicare because Medicare pays less than private health insurance.

We can't even agree as a country on the best way to protect ourselves from guns or the Coronavirus, or whether everyone is entitled to healthcare, paid family leave after a baby is born, or whether children born in our society are entitled to enough food, safe housing, adequate childcare, or education.

How are we going to agree on what the best healthcare should involve? This may be the most significant cost of racism to our whole society—a failure to do what is right for everybody means that no one gets the very best care.

Societies that trust their government and governmental agencies to manage crises did better in the pandemic because everyone pulled together, which is needed for public health to be effective.

In our divided society, we had groups of people asserting their right not to wear masks or get vaccinated, no matter who it hurt. President Trump even made resistance to public health measures political, so more Republicans died of COVID than Democrats who took precautions.

Sadly, those who benefit financially from the present system will resist change. Some medical providers may be moving toward getting big money out of medicine and adding more alternative, complementary, and holistic therapies, but others are buying up medical practices and hospitals in order to make more money.

Until we embrace a system that acknowledges all the advances that affect our health; all our knowledge of nutrition and exercise; and how food boosts the immune system and can prevent or reverse heart disease, diabetes, and cancer, we won't be doing the best we can for all sick people and our nation as a whole.

Until medical education includes natural therapies (including nutrition and exercise), we will be allowing the traditional weakness in our constitutional system to control healthcare rather than use this opportunity of massive national disruption to drive us to make positive changes for the practice of medicine.

Looking at the advances of the past fifty years, we can see that public health measures are most effective when the majority of people adhere to them. This includes actions on the part of individuals, medical practitioners, the food industry, the pharmaceutical industry, and especially the federal government.

Some see the federal government as the protector of business—American capitalism at work. Laws that interfere with or restrain trade can be easily overturned for that reason. Those in medicine have often used "restraint of trade" arguments to get their way. If someone can make money doing something, even if it does not benefit the community, it's very hard to stop them under our laws.

The American Medical Association has focused on *the business* of medicine and private insurance rather than the effectiveness of medicine and maximizing the health of the nation. But that was before American medicine became primarily a business, and doctors employed by the business were expected to make money by ordering the most tests and spending less time talking to patients.

Unfortunately, unless the federal government initiates policies to affect the whole population's health, any individual effort will be lacking.

In his book, *The China Study*, T. Colin Campbell tells the story of trying to bring his nutritional research to the attention of the appropriate government agencies, only to find that those agencies setting policies about our diet and food were run by representatives from the very industries out to make money from processed food. They would not even consider his research.

As long as we have government agencies dominated by business interests and not operating in the public's interest, we will have this problem.

When the treatment of African Americans under slavery and Jim Crow laws became too outrageous for the nation, Congress enacted legislation to outlaw such behaviors and policies. The Coronavirus pandemic exposed the flaws in our medical system.

In response, Congress could write laws mandating that medical schools teach nutrition, exercise, and some alternative therapies. Federal grant payments could be made contingent on compliance, but with the right will, this could be done. Such a policy would be the fastest way to galvanize change in this country since money always drives the engine here.

Gun Violence

SADLY, BOTH THE HOUSE and Senate are currently more focused on staying in power than fixing problems. Congress could also fund grants to medical schools to teach relevant public health topics and study the most effective way to deliver better health to the masses.

Among the public health issues that need to be addressed is gun safety, but again, like promoting business, unregulated gun use is a winning issue for Republicans running for office.

In 2017 alone, 39,773 people died because of gun violence, while over 100,000 were shot and injured. Assault weapons are not only more likely to kill and cause devastating injuries, but they can also be fitted with high-capacity magazines, allowing shooters to kill and maim more people in a short period of time. There is no legitimate reason to allow military-style weapons in the hands of the public. Shooting clubs for those who want to use these weapons could be licensed and monitored.

There are one or more mass shootings almost every day in the U.S. Children are growing up with mass-shooting drills while Congress refuses to act on the subject. Guns are now the biggest cause of death in the young. Every day, our children face the threat of being killed at school that day. States that have taken it upon themselves to enact gun regulations have lower rates of gun injuries and deaths. Alabama is second only to Alaska in the highest number of gun deaths. Louisiana is number three.[62]

We cannot deal with gun deaths without acknowledging our role as a nation in causing and supporting wars around the world for the last 30+ years. Supporting our gun industry and willingness to see adversaries everywhere has made us the "Big Satan." Plus, our failure to ratify the nuclear test ban treaty means we are back in a nuclear arms race. The U.S. has budgeted more than 634 billion to beef up its nuclear arsenal between 2021 and 2032[63]. This moves us closer to nuclear Armageddon all the time.

Public health should also include air and water quality, along with other environmental issues affecting health. Does Congress not see the climate crisis as a health issue? Extreme weather is already having profound health effects around the world.

In the coming decades, we will see climate migrants from

62　Don Johnson, Patch, "What Gun Violence Actually Looks Like in Alabama Lawmakers," October 2019. News outlets and high schoolers have their sights set on the AR-15. So, we decided to take a wider look at gun violence.

63　Kingston Reif &Sharon Bugg, from the Congressional Budget Office, June 2021. The Congressional Budget Office has estimated $756 billion for the nuclear arsenal between 2023-2032.

everywhere, even within our own country, as the dangers from fires, hurricanes, tornadoes, heat domes, and flooding continue to ravage the nation.

Opiates

WITH REGARD TO OPIATES, Congress needs to mandate a study on the so-called pain assessment, including the "fifth vital sign."

Officials should examine the use of the ten-point scale used to measure pain in hospital settings and mandate an alternative to training everyone to take pills when they hurt.

Congress could mandate that doctors be trained in the use of opiates and other drugs that can be abused and tested every five years to assess their understanding.

The current system demonstrates how ignorant, if not corrupt, current opiate prescribing practices appear to be. Opiates and other drugs that tend to be abused are best used to maximize function, not to be taken to feel better. This means prescribing more opiates when pain is highest. When pain decreases, they should only be used to help the patient function better and be more active.

Congress should also mandate that representatives from the food or pharmaceutical industries cannot staff the FDA. They should mandate guidelines that reflect current scientific knowledge about food, diet, the environment, and gun safety and not merely cater to the wishes of food manufacturers, polluters, and the NRA. Congress should also encourage a change in hospital diets through financial rewards or punishments under government contracts.

People everywhere in this country want policies that benefit themselves and their families. Congress needs to find a way to depoliticize the federal government's activities related to the nation's health. As long as health issues—such as guns, food, abortion, fossil fuels, etc.—are seen as a road to reelection, we won't have action.

Getting big money out of medicine is tricky and complicated, but until inexpensive natural methods like nutrition, exercise, meditation, etc., are part of general medical education and treatment, I think the best approach is to expand the education of the general public.

I still believe the great majority of doctors are not just out for the money but truly want what is best for their patients. They, like me, are concerned about the direction medicine has taken.

American Capitalism and Christianity

WE ARE NOW AT a crossroads where the cost of American capitalism has put the lives and health of our people on the line. The law, the constitution, and the whole political system are rigged in favor of money, the rich, business, political power, and racism. They're not designed to protect the poor, the sick, children, minorities, or the rest of us!

Surely, at this time when the pandemic has exposed systemic racism in the criminal justice system and shown us the downside of a racist healthcare system that favors profit for doctors, insurance companies, medical conglomerates, and Big Pharma over the health of the entire nation, isn't this the time to push for fundamental changes to the structure of government that will protect the most powerless in our midst?

Our system even protects climate deniers (or liars) who are getting rich off the fossil fuel industry and threatening our very existence on this planet.

Today, we see more people aware of our draconian history moving to support African Americans and Indigenous populations, plus the poor and working-class people. At the same time, we are seeing draconian measures to expand discrimination, interfere with voting rights, and deny beneficial programs to the poor and young.

I once believed that white Christian people were advocating for doing the right thing, but now it's clear that some white Christian churches have become the bastions of hate and violence against the rights of women, gays, blacks, and others, willing to use lies about our elections, our leaders and our institutions to win elections and stay in power. They are willing to undermine fair elections, dismantle democracy, and undermine the foundations of our government, aimed to protect us all, even waving the Bible as their guide.

If we are going to survive this onslaught on the message of Jesus and our Constitution, we need to find a way to become more inclusive and structurally change today's American capitalism into a more democratic capitalism like that of some Scandinavian countries—a system in which special interests or big money don't own the Supreme Court, and both houses of Congress so they can override attempts to level the playing field, and where finally a Christian approach is based on the admonition to love all our neighbors as ourselves.

Faced with endless challenges—global warming, overpopulation, massive worldwide migration, and endless pandemics and wars, etc.—that approach will better help us all to survive.

We could become a nation where even prisons become a place to educate those who have broken the laws, especially the unprotected young, so that they can live more productive lives.

But this won't happen unless we can finally see this nation's youth as everyone's responsibility to feed, educate, and protect. As a religious nation, we must remember the admonition of all religions, "Do unto others as you would have them do unto you."

As a psychiatrist privileged to observe human faults, foibles, and illnesses in all walks of life, I have seen how greed and selfishness have undermined the strength of our nation from its inception to the present.

In my next book, *Everybody's Nuts! Or Why Even Good People Do Terrible Things!* I explore the reasons human beings do the things they do and how to become more aware or mindful.[64]

---

64   Plague, the Black Death, Tuberculosis (TB), Syphilis and Chlamydia, Scarlet Fever, Measles, Mumps, Whooping Cough, Legionnaires' Disease.

Author's Comments and Acknowledgements

When I retired from the practice of medicine in 2005, I began writing two books: "Heal: A Psychiatrist's Inspiring Story of What it Takes to Recover from Chronic Pain, Depression, and Addiction...and What Stands in the Way" and "Heal Thyself: What You Can Do to Recover From Chronic Pain, Depression and Addiction." Both are self-published and available on Amazon.

Then in 2015 while my husband was writing a novel, I decided to write a story of what I had learned as a patient having MS since I was thirty years old. Armed with some notes on the folly my profession and what I had learned about what helped me survive MS, I began writing this book. This process has led me down many paths I had not anticipated at the beginning. I am grateful to many authors and researchers who expanded my world view in that process.

I am also grateful to my doctors and my patients who all added greatly to my understanding of how healing works and how we doctors might do it better. In addition, over the years I have had many great teachers to whom I owe a lot, among them Dr Abraham Russacoff, who showed in his approach to patients the importance of the doctor-patient relationship.

During thirty years of my practice, I lectured medical students about areas of psychiatry best understood by psychiatrists but usually practiced by internists and even surgeons. I talked about pain, depression, anxiety, addiction, and organic mental syndromes like delirium [confusion] and dementia. I'm grateful to my students who asked questions (or failed to ask questions) that expanded my understanding and knowledge of the limitations of doctors themselves and what needs to be changed in their practices.

A fourth book I continue to work on is, "Everybody's Nuts or Why Even Good People Do Terrible Things." I began collecting material for this from the moment I became a doctor in 1964. I have continued that practice through my more than forty years as a physician and psychiatrist. Part of the NUTS book is about the insanity I have observed in my profession.

I owe a special thanks to my sister, Anne Miller, who was most helpful in editing the book, having been a professional editor herself at one time. Thanks also to Christine Horner who skillfully edited, performed the layout, and created the cover. And I am indebted to members of my writing group, Fiction Critique, who shared their own work and feedback about what I was writing: David Roberts, Willum Fowler, Ron Carter, Barbara Powell, Paul Eleazor, and Larry Smith.

Finally, I'm grateful to my husband, Steve Coleman who took the writing journey with me while traveling to Northern Ireland for thirteen summers where I had time to write and think about what I wanted to say. There he read my material and listened to my thoughts as I tried to pour out my words of wisdom. In the end I would not have completed this book if it were not for Steve an accomplished writer and a very supportive husband who inspired and encouraged me throughout my efforts to create this book.

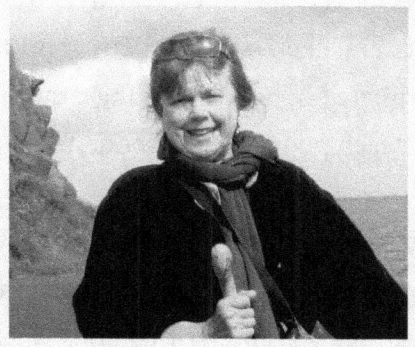

Author's Biography

SUMTER M. CARMICHAEL, MD is a retired board-certified psychiatrist living in Birmingham, Alabama with her husband, Steve Coleman. Dr. Carmichael graduated from Stanford University and completed her MD degree at Cornell University Medical College in New York City. Following a medical internship under Dr. Tinsley Harrison in Birmingham, she performed research at the Cardiovascular Research Center, Birmingham and at Virginia Heart Lab in Charlottesville. Returning to Birmingham for her psychiatric residency, she studied for seven years with a Freudian and a Jungian analyst.

After being diagnosed with Multiple Sclerosis, Dr, Carmichael opened a private practice, also working closely with a pastoral counseling center. She continued a hospital-based practice at University of Alabama-Birmingham, conducting individual, family, and group psychotherapy. In addition, she lectured to medical students in pharmacology and medicine.

In 1990 she began working with indigent medical

patients at the local county hospital, also teaching young doctors about pain, depression, anxiety, and addiction. This practice culminated in her developing a multidisciplinary pain clinic to teach poor patients about healing that comes from within.

Since her retirement and marriage to Steve Coleman, she has devoted her time to helping raise grandchildren, creating art, gardening, and writing books based upon her rich and varied professional experiences.

www.ingramcontent.com/pod-product-compliance
Lightning Source LLC
Chambersburg PA
CBHW070909130626
46555CB00001B/67